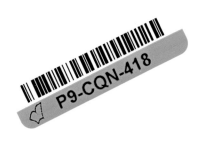

THE GIFT OF PETS

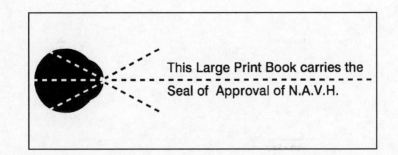

This Large Print Book carries the
Seal of Approval of N.A.V.H.

THE GIFT OF PETS

STORIES ONLY A VET COULD TELL

BRUCE R. COSTON, D.V.M.

THORNDIKE PRESS

A part of Gale, Cengage Learning

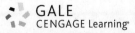

Detroit • New York • San Francisco • New Haven, Conn • Waterville, Maine • London

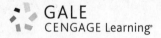
GALE
CENGAGE Learning®

Copyright © 2012 by Bruce R. Coston.
Thorndike Press, a part of Gale, Cengage Learning.

ALL RIGHTS RESERVED
Thorndike Press® Large Print Biography.
The text of this Large Print edition is unabridged.
Other aspects of the book may vary from the original edition.
Set in 16 pt. Plantin.

LIBRARY OF CONGRESS CIP DATA ON FILE:
CATALOGUING IN PUBLICATION DATA FOR THIS BOOK
IS AVAILABLE FROM THE LIBRARY OF CONGRESS

ISBN 13: 978-1-4104-5267-2 (hardcover)
ISBN 10: 1-4104-5267-0 (hardcover)

Published in 2012 by arrangement with St. Martin's Press, LLC.

Printed in the United States of America
1 2 3 4 5 6 7 16 15 14 13 12

In recognition of the grace she
displayed in meeting the
many challenges she faced,
for the courage she showed
in reinventing herself,
for her unswerving devotion
to the animals under her care,
and in memory of a short life well lived,
this book is lovingly dedicated to

Lisa Spalding, L.V.T.
(1963–2002)

CONTENTS

ACKNOWLEDGMENTS

There are many people involved in bringing these simple stories to you. The first are those wonderful and eclectic groups of people and animals who are the subjects of the stories. All of the stories are true, though some dialogue may be altered and some people may be composites of several actual clients. For those of you who may recognize yourself in the narrative, please know that it is with appreciation and respect that I relayed your part in the stories told.

I am very appreciative of my office staff for being unwitting subjects in the book. Susan, Rachel, and Krystal are still employees in the hospital and have been very gracious about their inclusion in the book. Rachel, who continues her April Fools' Day shenanigans (some of which have been cut from this memoir) got to choose her name in these pages. Susan, as of the spring of 2012, has worked with me in the office for twenty years, longer than many marriages.

Much gratitude goes to Lisa, though I cannot thank her personally, as you will see. I appreciate Lisa's family for letting me tell a story that may be difficult for them to read. Lisa's is a story of great courage and strength, of personal reinvention and professional growth. But it is also filled with sadness still for those who love her. Thank you, Amelia, Melanie, and Steven for allowing me to share her story with my readers.

I am greatly indebted to Cynthia, Jace, and Tucker for their patience with the process of writing this book. It was often a mistress that distracted me from family events. They are also featured in it, perhaps against their will. I love you all so very much and am grateful beyond words for each of you.

My agent, Jacques de Spoelberch, was a great help in honing and refining *The Gift of Pets* while keeping faith in its eventual success. He is to be credited for helping to keep a few stories in it that were slated for removal as too sad for animal lovers. When Simone passed, his faithful canine companion of many shared years and some 7,000 common miles, it was Jacques who argued that such sadness is a rich and valuable component of our lives with our pets. Even the sadness is a Gift, a testament to the depth of meaning they bring. Thank you, Jacques, for the assistance and professionalism you brought to this project.

A huge thank-you is extended to the entire team of wonderful professionals at Thomas Dunne Books. Toni Plummer has been a partner and active participant in bringing this book to you, and her skills, suggestions, and input have made it better than the manuscript she was originally presented. The copy editor, Carol Edwards, worked to improve the clarity and flow of the stories. And the cover designers, the typesetters, the publicity team, and the rest, whose names I don't even know, make the production and distribution of books seem seamless and simple, though I can see that it is not.

Finally, I thank my readers who respond so positively to the telling of these stories. Many, many letters, responses on my author Web site (www.brucecoston.com), e-mails, and comments at book events have come my way, and they highlight how deep is the impact our animals have on our hearts. Thank you for reading these stories. Go ahead . . . tell your friends!

PROLOGUE: THE HARVEYS

I envy the Harvey children. There are four siblings in the Harvey family, stair-stepped, when I first met them, from age seven to about age twelve. I have trouble keeping them all straight, since I see them only four or five times a year and seldom all together. They insist upon continuing to grow, so I often apply the wrong name to the wrong child. You would know instantly if you saw them that they are siblings, since they all look very much alike. The four are home-schooled and therefore are their own best friends. The Harveys are a close family. It's evident in the way they interact with one another and with their mother, Danielle. But that's not the reason I envy them.

The reason is that the Harvey family is perhaps the most animal-oriented family I have ever served. Numbering among the Harvey pets I have treated are two dogs, four cats, two guinea pigs, a gerbil, a rat, and the most responsive bird I have ever known. And there are those I have not treated on their small homestead: horses, goats, geese, and, no doubt, others. What I would have given to have been able to indulge my animal passion similarly when I was growing up! But alas, I was born to parents who shared not a single animal-loving gene between them. Don't get me wrong. I'm not complaining, just reporting. Two Harvey patients I have treated spring to mind.

Collin was about nine or ten when I first met him. He is a quiet young man with little to say to strangers like me. He has dark hair, a large round face, and an impish grin. Despite his quiet demeanor, I suspect there are levels of mischief in him that were not evident as he sat quietly in my exam room.

What was immediately apparent when I walked in for our first introduction was the abiding bond between Collin and the diminutive bird he cradled protectively in his hand. Parrots are universally suspicious creatures, convinced that all newcomers are dangerous predators. This is an important survival strategy for them in the wild, where such a presupposition can be lifesaving. But virtually all birds bring this attitude to every veterinary interaction, hopping quickly around their cages, carefully keeping as much space as possible between themselves and me, their heads cocking and attentive to every movement or sound I make.

Not so with Precious, Collin's little Black-Capped Conure. Precious was not in a cage at all! Instead, she was cuddled serenely on Collin's chest as he slouched like a teenager against the wall, his hands cupped around her and his fingers lovingly caressing the feathers around her face. Though she looked at me and fluffed her feathers nervously when I entered the room, she stayed in the safety of his hand and chortled quietly. Collin gently raised her from his chest and turned her over onto her back so she was lying feet-up in his open palms. With his thumbs, he smoothed the feathers on her belly from her throat to her legs. I expected Precious to squawk and struggle at this indignity, as most birds would do in the strange surroundings of a veterinary hospital. But to my amazement, she closed her eyes, clubbed her little feet into fists, and went soundly to sleep. I was astonished! I had seen few animals do this in my office, much less a bird. The trust she placed in Collin was truly unique, and I was enormously impressed.

Precious has been a joy to treat over the

years, not least because she has been a very healthy bird, thanks to the wonderful care Collin provides her. A part of his home schooling has been to familiarize himself with the best diet and husbandry practices for her species, and this has resulted in the ideal diet and care for her. So far, the only treatments she has required have been routine trimming of her toenails, wings, and beak. These she has submitted to with patience and dignity, always attended by her special friend, Collin.

Much has changed for Collin since I first met him. He is taller and more mature. His home situation has changed. Even his voice has changed. As he grew, I wondered whether the mounting insecurities of adolescence might diminish his willingness to invest the same degree of emotion and attentiveness in his friend. But despite all the other changes in his life, his devotion to Precious remains the same, an anchor in his world to the firm, unchanging realities that are undiminished by advancing time. For Collin, Precious has been precious indeed.

Collin's little brother, Evan, looks very much like his big brother. But there the similarities end. Whereas Collin's personality runs quiet and deep, Evan's is a babbling brook, splashing and rapid and continuously moving. This is not to suggest that he is shallow; far from it. The same amount of water flows through the rapids as the deep, quiet pools. It's just the rate of flow that changes. Evan is a whir of frenetic activity and fun. He is quick with a joke and a laugh and eager to engage in conversation.

Evan, like Collin, had a special pet. Her name was Gabby, and she was a two-and-a-half pound rat with short white hair and a long scaly tail. She measured easily two feet from the tip of her nose to the end of her reptilian tail. Her nose protruded ahead of her and bent downward at the tip, with long whiskers that constantly moved. She had two long yellowed incisors that protruded from her busy little mouth. If you looked at Gabby with the prejudices that are typically directed at rats, she was a conniving, vile, disease-carrying vermin. But if you looked at her through Evan's eyes, she was a sweet, responsive, intelligent, curious, and much-loved pet.

Handling Gabby did make you reconsider your assumptions about the species. I found her to be a gentle, inquisitive, and thoroughly enjoyable little animal. It was clear from the way she and Evan interacted that they had developed a relationship of mutual trust and appreciation. If for no other reason, this special bond deserved my full attention to Gabby's health.

There are no routine rat vaccines that bring these pets to the veterinarian annually. We see rats when there is a health issue that needs attention. I first met Gabby when Evan, then about eight years old, and Danielle brought her in to have me evaluate a lump that had developed under her white skin. I was surprised at the extent of the lump as I examined her on the table, Evan looking on with concern. It started at about the midline on her belly and extended up her side halfway to her backbone. It was firm and painless, but it was so large that it interfered with Gabby's ability to walk normally, as it would have mine had an anvil been implanted under the skin on my side. In all other respects, Gabby appeared completely normal.

I knew what this growth was right away, having seen similar cases and read about them in the veterinary literature. This was a tumor of the breast tissue, which in the rat extends well up the sides. Because it was a fast-growing mass, I suspected it was malignant. The best hope would be for me to remove the growth surgically. While this was unlikely to effect a cure, it would at least extend Evan's time with Gabby and make her more comfortable in the interim. I turned to discuss my findings with the Harveys, being careful to direct my comments not to Danielle but to Gabby's owner.

"Evan," I began. "I really don't like the looks of that growth. How long have you noticed it?"

"It's been probably three or four weeks," he said uncertainly, looking at his mother for confirmation. She nodded.

"And how old is Gabby now?"

"I think she's about four years old," he responded. Danielle nodded her head again.

"Well, Evan," I continued, "I think this growth is a tumor of the milk-producing cells in Gabby."

Evan nodded solemnly. I suspected his mother had prepared him for this possibility. "Does that mean cancer?"

"I think so, Evan. I can't say for sure without a biopsy, but most of these types of growths in rats are cancerous." I watched as his eyes filled with concern and tears. "I'm so sorry. I know that makes you sad, doesn't it?"

"Is there anything we can do for her?"

"Our best hope is to do surgery as soon as possible to remove the growth. I doubt the surgery will cure her, but it will make it easier for her to move around and give her longer to live than she would have if we didn't do it."

"How long would she live without surgery?"

"I suppose at the rate this has grown, she would live another three to six weeks. If we do surgery, I think we could increase that to maybe three to six months."

Evan turned hopeful eyes to his mother at my words. There was a plea on his face that required no words. Danielle cocked her head at him in warning before she spoke.

"Evan, you remember we talked about this before we came here today. We knew this is what Dr. Coston might say. I suppose surgery will be an expensive option, and we need to be realistic about the decisions we make."

Evan's head fell and he wiped a tear from his cheek. Meekly, he turned to me. "About how much would it cost to do the surgery?"

"Your mother is right, Evan. It would be relatively expensive. I'll have to get the hospital manager to estimate the costs for me. Surgery is a relatively costly endeavor, though. Are you sure you want me to figure that out?"

Evan's face turned resolute and hopeful at my question, perhaps even a bit indignant.

Who was I to question his commitment to his pet on the sole basis of monetary considerations? "I have some money in the bank I've been saving for a new bicycle. I could use it for Gabby's surgery instead. She's my responsibility, you know, and I love her."

"That's very kind of you, Evan. I'll be glad to prepare an estimate for the surgery. Give me just a few minutes."

I left Gabby with Evan and his mother and went into Susan's office, knowing that the discussion between them would continue in my absence. Susan and I put together an estimate for the surgery that kept the costs to as low a figure as we possibly could. It included the materials and the supplies but did not include any profit from the procedure. I'd already appreciated a healthy return on the transaction in seeing Evan's fierce determination to help his untraditional pet.

I felt certain that the process of developing a cost estimate was an exercise in futility. When the costs of a procedure like this are weighed against the costs of replacing a rat, the rational thing to do is to replace the rat. That's obvious. I had seen these cases before, but seldom had a client elected to invest money in the surgery. I can't honestly say that I blame these clients. After all, finances are a real and valid consideration. I am not so naïve as to think otherwise. The question I am tempted to ask the client in these cases is, "Do you want *a* rat or do you want *this* rat? Though it may seem an insensitive question, when it came right down to it, practically every client I had dealt with in this same situation had chosen reason over emotion. I suspected the same would be true for Evan and Danielle.

"It looks like the costs for this surgery will be a little over a hundred and fifty dollars, Evan," I said after returning to the room. "But depending on how things go and how long it takes, it could be as much as a couple hundred dollars." Danielle's head snapped up and she looked me in the eyes, her face perplexed. She knew my estimate was ridiculously low for the degree of effort involved. Slowly, a look of deep appreciation settled on her face as she turned again to Evan.

"That's less than we had anticipated," she said. "Evan, I know you have seventy-five dollars saved up that you want to spend on Gabby. I'm willing to help out some, too. But this will mean that you'll have to use your allowance for a while to pay for this. Are you sure you want to do that?"

Evan nodded emphatically. There was no

hesitation in his response, no reluctance to commit his own money to the care of his friend, even knowing it was unlikely to effect a cure. It was a level of commitment and responsibility that I wish all my clients displayed.

That afternoon, I anesthetized Gabby and performed the first and only rat mastectomy of my twenty-three-year veterinary career. With extreme care, I dissected away the invading mass from Gabby's side. It was a technically demanding procedure because the size of my patient, though large for a rat, was much smaller than the typical animal that went under my knife. It was difficult, too, because the tumor had woven itself around Gabby's normal anatomical features. But mostly, it was demanding because throughout the hour-long procedure I was constantly cognizant of the close communion between this animal and the little boy sitting, worried and impatient, by the phone. And I was reminded again that even the relationships that I didn't necessarily understand had inestimable value to those whose hearts were hopelessly enmeshed within them.

Later that evening, I sent Gabby home to one very excited little boy. I fashioned a collar from used X-ray film, similar to the collars placed on dogs and cats to prevent the licking of wounds. Rats are notorious for their obsessive attention to suture lines. I did not want Gabby to chew out the neat row of stitches I had placed. She looked more than funny with a miniature inverted lamp shade over her head. I teased Evan, saying that she should come back in two weeks to have her stitches removed and her lightbulb changed.

Gabby healed beautifully. She left her stitches alone during the two weeks the collar was in place, and the surgical wound healed; only the slightest of scars remained, bearing witness to the surgery she had undergone. Though she did later succumb to the breast cancer, the end was forestalled for many months and Evan enjoyed his additional time with her. When she did pass away, I sent my customary letter of condolence to him and included this touching poem by Ruby King Phillips.

Today
I said goodbye to a friend
Though there can be no end
To all he was to me.
With one last sigh
He drifted into sleep
And I was left to keep

Intact the gifts he gave. . . .
Eyes, warm and grave
That almost speak,
Small furry paw
Against my cheek,
Faithful presence
Always there beside my chair. . . .
Loyalty and utmost trust
Perish not nor turn to dust.
Beyond the cosmic reach of earth
Where only Love can be
Where Time cannot be measured
I know he's running free.

Relationships between people and their pets are intensely personal ones and greatly enhance the emotional richness of both the people and their devoted animals. These human-animal bonds can be some of the most profound interactions we humans engage in. Something about the unfounded trust our pets place in us, the singleness of their devotion, their unrestrained joy in simply being with us, and the indifference with which they regard our flaws makes their companionship incomparable. We become better people because of the way they see us.

The interface between people and pets is one of the few interactions where we can comprehend what it means to be emotionally involved and readily available to another being; to be dependent upon, yet strengthened by, something outside ourselves. Paradoxically, loving a pet teaches us to be fully human.

Unfortunately, not everyone experiences the ennobling effects of animals. Not every heart is tugged by the intensity of love in the eyes of a noble graying canine or feline face. This is completely inexplicable to me. I have come to understand that it is a Gift to be blessed with this passion for animals; a Gift that all who share it understand innately, and that those without it can never comprehend.

It is at the intersection between animals and those people who possess the Gift that we veterinarians spend our professional lives. Exploring the intimacies of the human-animal bond is what brings meaning and value to what we do. It is a rare privilege indeed to invest our lives so completely in the Gift. For we are privy to some of the most touching stories of love and devotion that exist — stories that evoke the most noble of human emotions, that plumb the deepest of human motives; stories that inspire us, amuse us, challenge us, or cause tears to spring unbidden to our eyes.

Evan has grown up quite a bit since then. He remains the bright and engaging young man I first met many years ago and continues to enjoy his relationship with the more traditional of the family pets that I still see routinely. He has not since fallen in love with another rat, as far as I know. But one thing I do know. He will never look back on his time with Gabby and have regrets. He will not have to think with remorse about the time his mother and his vet minimized the value of a relationship they did not share or understand. Perhaps someday, that memory will stimulate a similar response to the whimsical passions of his own children — and the circle will have been completed.

I may have seen the Harveys for the last time a couple of weeks back. Since I first started seeing their menagerie some years ago, the fortunes of the Harveys have dramatically changed. A series of unfortunate events has left them reeling. Danielle is planning on moving her children to a new community to start over. As of yet, they have not selected where that place will be. But it most likely will not be near enough to our practice to allow them to continue bringing their dwindling animal crew to see me. I will miss them.

But I will carry much of value from my association with them. I will always treasure the interactions I am blessed to have with families as a whole, and with the children of those families in particular. I will be reminded to validate every precious human-animal relationship, even if I don't share the passion. And I will bring my best to every patient because such a love demands my best.

Though they have faced difficult circumstances, the Harvey children will emerge from Danielle's home with at least one wonderful legacy. They will have learned that to love animals is a blessing to be cherished; that having pets is a responsibility one must take seriously and for which one is rewarded with loyalty and trust. They have experienced the wonder of bonding with an individual of a different order, with whom communication occurs on levels far deeper than mere words, where the ties are stronger than time, and where the rewards are not measured by how much can be reciprocated by an animal but by how much we are willing to invest. These valuable life lessons are best learned under the tutelage of animals, for they are not contaminated by the same innate self-interest that corrupts many human relationships.

The Harvey kids have grown up with the Gift: the Gift of valuing animals; of loving a pet so wholly that the ache at parting is indelibly insinuated into their futures; of receiving devotion untainted by duplicity; of experiencing unequaled loyalty and unveiled adoration. This Gift is a birthright that I share with the Harvey children.

It is the Gift that for my whole life has guided my education, informed my decisions, and determined my career path. It is the Gift that has surrounded me with orphaned blue jays and squirrels, with parakeets, hamsters, dogs, cats, and cockatiels. It is the Gift that has tasked me with not only a profession but a passion — a mission. Obeying the directives of the Gift has at times been demanding and emotionally excruciating. But it has also afforded a life of unequaled satisfaction and amazing fulfillment. The rewards that come with seeing the face of one like Evan fill with joy and relief at the reunion with a recovered pet cannot be understood without firsthand experience. But as a veterinarian, those undeserved rewards accrue to me daily.

The Gift of Pets is, for me, a defining reality. I'm not sure who I would be in its absence. I could not survive without it, nor would I want to. I suspect you know of what I speak. The fact that you are reading this probably means you, too, share it. Countless people are born with the Gift, as I was. Many have nurtured and developed this genetic bequest, allowing it to blossom into wonderful fruition. But few have been raised within it like the Harveys. It is for this blessing that I envy them.

Mountain of Love

I watched with interest as Mr. Johnston escorted his bullmastiff into the waiting room. This would have been an effort at any time because of the sheer bulk of the patient. But progress was made all the more difficult by the massive growth encasing the beast's upper thigh, rendering the right hind leg nearly useless. As the dog made her way through the door and down the hall, awkwardly swinging her leg wide and hunching her back in order to lift the leg and advance the foot just a few inches forward, the knee remained fixed and rigid, forcing the toes to scrape the ground as slow progress was made. Traversing the length of the twenty-foot hallway consumed nearly two minutes. Finally, with the help of the technician and the encouragement of the owner, she made her way onto the scale. The digits on the digital display danced for a bit before settling at 165 pounds.

In the examination room, I surveyed both the patient and her owner. Mr. Johnston was unique. Only about five feet six inches or so, he must have weighed more than three hundred pounds. In order to fit all that mass into such a small frame, his contour sported bulges around his center, making him seem almost as round as he was tall. His strawlike yellow hair was long, billowing, and wild, as if the trip over the pass from Fort Valley had been made with his head out the open window. He kept sweeping this hair up and back over his head with his hand as clutches of the stuff broke free and fell like coils of baling twine across his forehead, obscuring his eyes. His cheeks and nose were puffy and red and streaked like a city map with a network of prominent veins. His lower eyelids drooped sadly, Basset-like, a puff of pillowed and pale skin hanging loosely like dusty drapes below each of them. His upper lids seemed a bit too heavy to keep fully open, forcing him to tilt his head back slightly to turn his eyes up to my face.

He was dressed in dark sweatpants, the waist of which was cinched tightly around his middle, the drawstring dimpling his tummy at that spot, with adipose tissue bulging several inches above and below the knot. I hoped the drawstring was strong. I was sure that if it broke free, the pants would soon be around his ankles. I did not indulge the mental image. At the end of his legs, the pants failed to reach the white high-topped tennis shoes he wore, this probably owing to the degree to which he'd had to hitch the front of the pants up to cover his girth. Above his waistline, he wore a buttoned-up dress shirt, the bottom of which just swept the top of the sweatpants. It accommodated his girth only by his having left the last buttons undone. The effect was to make both the shirt and the pants seem ridiculously incongruous.

"Hello, Mr. Johnston. How are you this morning?"

"I'm fine. It's Dahmun I'm worried about." He got right to the point.

"What's her name?" I had never encountered one quite like it.

"It's Dahmun!" He offered no further explanation, but after a short pause, he spelled it as if for a dim-witted schoolboy. "D-A-H-M-U-N." He shook his head and clucked his tongue in annoyance.

"Where did you get that name?"

Mr. Johnston exhaled an impatient sigh, as if my question was delaying some more important engagement.

"Well, among other things, I'm a linguist." He paused in order to let the significance of that sink in. "The name is a patented syllylogy."

I stared at him blankly. I had never encountered a syllylogy before, patented or otherwise, and my mind immediately veered dangerously into wondering with which government agency one would patent a syllylogy — or why.

"I have invented a language in which each syllable represents a discreet meaning. Words are then assembled which convey specific meaning by their very construction."

"So what does Dahmun mean, then?" I asked.

"Well, the syllables represent . . . I mean 'dah' is a . . . uh . . . a large landmass, especially one with lots of altitude. Combine that with the syllable 'mun,' which signifies deep affection and fondness. See?"

He looked at me, apparently to watch the light of meaning dawn in my foggy eyes. The fog persisted.

"No, I don't quite get your drift."

He clicked his tongue again, clearly impatient with the obvious dullness of the pupil before him.

"Dah-mun. Dah-mun. Get it? It literally

means 'Mountain of Love.' "

"Oh, I see now." And I really did begin at that moment to understand Mr. Johnston.

"Tell me what's been going on with Dahmun. Start at the very beginning, please."

"About four or five months ago, we were hiking on my property in the Fort."

Fort Valley is a blind valley with an open mouth on the north end. It is contained by two ridges that run along the east and west flanks of its fifteen- or twenty-mile length. The floor of the valley is no more than two or three miles at its widest and is choked off as the ridges squeeze together and finally join at the southern end. It's said that George Washington had scouted out this "fort valley" as a place to hide had the Revolutionary War gone badly. The valley would probably be missed if scouted either from the east or the west, and the mouth could be easily defended against intruders from the north. Over time, Fort Valley became the accepted name of the valley. It also became a place where lots of people settled who liked to hide their homes from prying eyes. It is occupied today by folks for whom Woodstock is too populated and occupied by weekenders escaping from the rush of the nation's capital. Locals call it simply "the Fort."

"Dahmun loves to go hiking with me. That day, we were going up a rather steep hill with loose gravel. She slipped and fell down on her poobus. I —"

"Excuse me." I interrupted him. I was carefully writing down the history in the record and was sure I had been concentrating too hard on this task to have heard him correctly. "What was it that she hit when she fell?"

"Her poobus!" He waited for me to catch up. My face was apparently broadcasting that I was helplessly clawing for clarity.

"Poobus. Poo-bus," he said again for me, more slowly this time and louder. I suspected another patented syllylogy, until he clapped his hand over the lower reaches of his right fanny and repeated again, "Poo-bus."

"Got it. Go on," I said, finally recognizing that he had just badly mangled the anatomical term *pubis.*

"So after she fell, she displayed some dysmobility for a few days. It might have lasted as long as a couple of weeks. Then it seemed to improve again. I wasn't too worried at that point. I just assumed she had pulled a muscular infraction or something. But then I noticed that the muscles in the right rear were beginning to atrophatize."

36

The linguistic license Mr. Johnston displayed began to tickle me. It seemed important to him that I recognize the mastery he possessed over nearly correct medical terminology. The oddities of the syntax and the reinvention of the words were so strange that I knew I would never remember them or be believed when I related them again. So I discreetly slid the record over and began to jot down on a sheet of paper towel the words he was inventing — *dysmobility, atrophatize.* This was good!

"Please go on, Mr. Johnston."

"About that time, I noticed that a lump was beginning to form at the top of the leg. It didn't really seem painful at the time. But over a period of several months, it's gotten bigger and bigger, until I thought I ought to have it checked out. It has also begun to cause her some pain. I'm sure it's just an abcleft. How much will you charge to have it lanceted?"

"I think it's a little early to talk about treatment," I responded. "I haven't even examined her yet. Let's take a look."

Dahmun was much too large to place on the examination table, so I began my exam by getting down on the floor with her. I started at the head and examined her eyes, ears, and nose. I then opened her cavernous mouth and inspected her bear-size teeth, tonsils, and tongue. My hands traced the lines of her neck, carefully outlining the lymph nodes, salivary glands, and trachea. All looked and felt normal. I heard an audible sigh again and looked up at Mr. Johnston.

"Doctor, the problem is not up there. The problem is back in the hind leg, see?" He rolled his eyes, as if I was too simple to recognize his unmistakable disdain.

"Yes, I noticed that when you came in the door. But you don't want me to miss something else important because I focused in too quickly on what was blatantly obvious, do you?"

He didn't answer. Apparently, he didn't care what I might miss. I continued my examination by listening intently to the dog's heart and the lungs. Then carefully, using both hands on her prodigious belly, I palpated the urinary bladder, the intestines, the kidneys, the spleen, and a bit of the liver poking beyond the arches of the last ribs. All seemed fine.

I then turned my attention to the leg. As Dahmun stood patiently, the toes on her right foot turned under and her leg was stocked in a taut straight line. The skin over her knees and toes bulged with swelling. At the top of her leg, by the hip, a huge mass, larger than a cantaloupe and as firm, encased the bone. The slightest pressure on this mass caused Dahmun to whine and squeal in pain. A little more pressure induced her to turn and nip at my hand apologetically.

I shook my head absently. This wasn't good. I turned and began to write my findings in the record, using this time to organize my thoughts around how I was going to discuss the problem with Mr. Johnston. Apparently, I was taking too long for him.

"So, now that you've had a chance to examine her, how much will you charge to lancet the abcleft?"

"I'm afraid lancing an abscess is not what we need to do here, Mr. Johnston." I sighed. I dislike being the bearer of bad news. But in this case, there was no other option. "The lump is not an abscess. Dahmun has a tumor in her leg. It entirely encases the femur just below the hip. It also apparently has the sciatic nerve entrapped within it, too. That's why she can't bend her leg, and why she knuckles over on her toes like that."

Mr. Johnston processed this for a moment. It was clear that he did not want to believe me.

"What is the causality of this problem?"

"I wish I could answer that question, Mr. Johnston. If we had the answer to why cancer occurs, we would be far along the road to its cure. But for most cancer types, we really haven't identified any specific cause-and-effect relationships. It's just one of those things that happen."

"Could it be the initial injury? Or is it un-expectable for an injury like that to cause tumors?"

"No. I suspect the injury was a result of the cancer, not the other way around. The tumor in its early stages may have made her unstable and led to the fall."

"And the swelling? Is that just the phle-bum that can't reticulate back up the leg?"

"Exactly," I agreed. "Because of the poor lymphatic return, extracellular fluid accumulates and causes that type of swelling. It's called 'pitting edema,' and it's a common consequence of such an invasive growth."

"I'm sure you're a good vet and all, Doctor. But I'm still not convinced this isn't just an abcleft. Can't you do some tests or something to find out?"

"Of course, Mr. Johnston. I'll do an aspiration cytology. I'll stick a needle into the tumor and draw some cells out that I can look at under the microscope. If this is just an abscess, what we'll get is pus. X-rays will also be very helpful in this case. But . . ." I shook my head to underscore my pessimism. "I'd love to be wrong here, Mr. Johnston. But I really don't think it's reasonable to expect that."

"You'll forgive me for this, but I'm eternally optometric."

I plunged a needle deep into the mass and could feel grating against the tip of the needle as I did so. The tumor had begun to incorporate calcium deposits into its structure — not a good sign. I then sprayed the contents of the needle onto a glass slide and took it to the laboratory. While the technicians took Dahmun to get X-rays of the swollen leg, I placed the slide under the microscope's lens. Peering through the eyepieces, I examined the cells I had collected. They were grossly abnormal.

Soon I was called into the radiology room to evaluate the X-rays. The films were classic for bone cancer. Feeling defeated, I trailed back into the exam room.

I came right to the point. "I'm afraid there is really no question about it." "The cells that I collected show all the telltale signs of cancer. And judging by the cellular characteristics, it looks to be quite an aggressive tumor at that. When we combine that with the textbook pattern I see on the X-rays, I'd say I'm more than ninety-five percent sure it's bone cancer. I'm so sorry. A definitive diagnosis can only be made by a pathologist examining a tissue section, but a biopsy confirmation wouldn't change our treatments much."

Mr. Johnston was quiet for a moment, absorbing the impact of my findings.

"It's my own fault. I should have brought her in earlier. I shouldn't have been so delaysive in getting her some help. What do we do now?"

"Well, I'm afraid there aren't many options at this point. These types of tumors don't respond very well to chemotherapy alone. In order to give her any chance at all, we would need to amputate the leg first, then follow with chemotherapy. This treatment has resulted in the best outcomes. One of the problems with that, though, is her size. She may not get around well at one hundred and sixty-five pounds with only three legs. It is also very likely that it has already spread to other areas."

"You think this has already metatheclized?" Mr. Johnston gasped.

"I don't know for sure. But it's very likely. The odds are very much against us. In order to know, we'd need to x-ray the chest and the abdomen and consider ultrasounding the belly." Sometimes you are beaten even before you begin the fight. And this was likely one of those cases.

"Perhaps the best thing for us to do is control her pain with medications for as long as we can. There are a number of ways we can do that."

Mr. Johnston sadly took his big Mountain of Love home. Prescription pain medications kept Dahmun's discomfort at bay for a few more weeks. But eventually, even those were inadequate to allay her constant suffering. As the bulbous growth enlarged ever more quickly, her ability to get up and move around declined precipitously. Soon there was nothing for us to do but ease her suffering in the most permanent of ways.

Mr. Johnston's loss was a difficult one, and I felt bad for him. But the episode apparently bolstered his confidence in me. Though he continues to exhibit the same disgusted frustration with me that he did when I first met Dahmun, he has presented several of his animals to me since then. I've learned some things about dealing with him. First, I never ask for explanations of the names he gives his pets. Second, I'll never go into the exam room again without a slip

43

of paper under the record to write down the lingering linguistic lapses.

THE CONTRACT

Greco was an interesting mixture of canine breeds. Somewhere in his distant past, there was certainly beagle blood. That much was clear. Beyond that, breeds and bloodlines blurred. Weighing in at about forty-five pounds, Greco sported the beagle colors but displayed the body contours of a shepherd. His attitude of braggadocio was clearly independent of his questionable lineage. The set of the tail, the carriage of the proud head, and the careless, almost disdainful persona stated with clarity, "I am who I am. I don't care who my ancestors weren't. I am *the* Greco." You had to like a dog like that. And Greco was quite confident that you would.

Greco's owner, Antonio Toumopoulis, seemed equally incongruous. His jet black hair, heavy eyebrows, dark skin, and deep Greek accent were unexpected deviations from the characteristic western Virginia drawl. Nonetheless, Mr. Toumopoulis bore these Greek characteristics with obvious pride. No apologies were necessary and none was proffered. He more than compensated for his diminutive five-foot-three stature by booming out his staccato dialogue in unbelievably amplified tones. The pair was indeed an impressive duo.

The visit that morning, though still carried on at rather uncomfortable decibel levels, was relatively suppressed. Greco was sick!

"Greco . . . he no feela good," Mr. Toumopoulis reported, endlessly rolling his *r*'s in ways that I can not force my tongue to imitate, much less represent in print. "Seence two day ago, he no eeta . . . no dreenka . . . no, how you say, poo." At least half of his meaning was evident from creative use of hand, arm, and facial gestures, which, in this context, are best not described. "And he . . . [more expressive gesturing] "breenga ohp hees fooda meeny time."

"Do you know of anything he could have gotten into? Any missing toys or things like that?" I queried, concerned about a possible gastrointestinal obstruction.

"Oh no, Doctohr. He no playa weeth toys. He theenka squeaky things too seessy. He more like chewa de rocks."

Stoically, Greco stood as if planted on my examination table. Too macho to exhibit his discomfort overtly, he simply stared straight ahead, eyes fixed on the wall in front of him. In response to hearing his name, he would give three or four tentative wags of the tail before assuming once again his statuesque pose. There was a barely noticeable catch in his throat as he drew each breath. Otherwise, he masked his discomfort completely.

I carefully felt his stomach with my fingers, gently probing the bladder, the spleen, the liver, and the intestines for any abnormalities. As I did so, I felt a golf ball–size lump slip through my fingers. When I bumped up against the firm lump, Greco's pain broke through his stoicism. He turned and snapped at my hand, barely missing, then immediately wagged his tail ingratiatingly, as if to say, "Sorry, Doc. But man, that hurt!"

I carried Greco to the X-ray room, where he bravely submitted to having pictures taken. A stark white object stood out as if in relief at one end of a dark tubular shadow in the abdominal cavity. Greco did indeed like to "chewa de rocks." This one was obstructing his bowel, trapping gas behind it, and painfully ballooning the intestines. I knew that surgery would be necessary.

I set Greco back on the examination table. He immediately resumed his painful posture, staring at the wall as if engrossed in must-see TV. I turned to Mr. Toumopoulis.

"The X-rays show an intestinal foreign body — probably a rock. It means we should go in surgically and remove it. I don't think this should wait. I'd like to do the surgery right away." I could see Mr. Toumopoulis's dark eyes flare with concern for his friend and suspicion of me.

"Ju theenka he need be cut hopen?"

"Yes, I do."

"He be hokay?"

"Not without surgery. And the sooner the better."

He eyed me uncertainly, apparently convinced of neither my diagnosis nor my capabilities. Finally: "Ju do thees . . . cutting before?"

"Yes, I have, Mr. Toumopoulis." I tried to be as reassuring as possible while at the same time maintaining a healthy realism. This was a serious condition and the risks were very real. "You must understand that Greco is seriously ill, and though it's unlikely, it's possible we could lose him during surgery. But without it, we'll lose him for sure."

Mr. Toumopolis studied the floor for a few moments, his dark eyebrows furrowed, almost meeting in the middle over his prominent nose. His hand ran over Greco's head, absently tracing the dog's forehead and ears. Greco didn't respond to his touch.

In the end, it wasn't my urging that finally convinced Mr. Toumopolis. It was Greco's quiet grunt of discomfort that brought him around. With a conflicted mixture of resignation and conviction, he turned to face me.

"Hokay, Doctohr. Ju go do cutting now. I waita for ju to call." He turned to go.

"Mr. Toumopoulis!" I stammered out too quickly. "There's something else."

When it comes to my practice, I hate more than anything the need to discuss the financial aspects of treating my patients. Human physicians, understandably, do not have to contend with financial constraints in the treatment of their patients. Veterinarians, on the other hand, are accustomed to these considerations and are always prepared to include financial matters in their discussions about treatment. Throughout my entire career, I have understood the importance of communicating clearly the expected costs of treatment. Few people are situated financially such that these discussions are unnecessary.

49

Strangely, it is perhaps these discussions that have made it possible — necessary, in fact — for the veterinary profession to remain the best value in the field of health care. In human medicine, with a massive percentage of costs accrued within the last weeks of life, including incredibly expensive diagnostic testing and budget-busting pharmaceuticals, costs have escalated exponentially — costs that are largely invisible to those who actually receive the services.

This is not so in veterinary medicine. Costs for care are borne directly by the ones who must make the decisions about health care. And each individual must consider the costs and the wider implications of those costs on families and loved ones. These factors have forced us to keep the costs for significantly sophisticated care to a fraction of those for similar human care. This is true even though the costs to a veterinary practitioner of providing services are higher than those for the typical family-practice physician. While physicians can refer their patients to the local hospital for X-rays, blood work, a sonogram, surgery, and hospitalization, we veterinarians must provide those capabilities in our offices and still somehow keep the costs manageable for the clients.

I turned to Mr. Toumopolis with resignation, knowing this part of the discussion was never fun.

"You need to know that surgery could be fairly expensive. For some people, that is a consideration. The business office can give you an estimate for the fees and arrange payment options if necessary. So I'll need you to —"

My words were interrupted by a flash of unhappiness in Antonio's dark eyes. "No . . . No . . . No . . ." Each word was punctuated by the jabbing of a thick finger in my chest. Then Antonio's eyes lightened and he addressed me in a rhythmic, almost musical cadence. "I tella ju vhat. Ju teka de responsibility to fixa de dohg; I teka de responsibility to paya de bill."

And that pretty much settled it. I accepted his terms and began work on my patient. Greco was hospitalized, and a large catheter was placed in his leg, through which we pumped fluids into his vein. His head sank in sleep as I pushed the anesthetic into the catheter before slipping a large plastic tube into his trachea, which allowed me to control his breathing and provide the anesthetic gas.

During surgery, I removed a man-size rock, which Greco had consumed during his macho play. It had lodged fast in the

51

small intestine, obstructing the passage of all gastrointestinal contents. The section of intestine containing the stone, now stretched and bruised to a dark purple, had sustained irreparable damage and had to be removed. But after an hour and a half of tedious suturing, I pulled the gloves off my hands and surveyed the neat row of sutures closing the eight-inch-long incision on Greco's tummy. Surgery had gone well and I was confident that Greco would recover fully.

No sooner had Greco opened his eyes after surgery than he was trying to stand. Within another ten minutes, he was staggering drunkenly toward the door. His sentiments and intentions were unmistakable. "Thanks, Doc," he was saying. "You did good. I'll take it from here. See ya later." We literally had to tie him down till he was fully recovered.

Greco went home the next day, much earlier than most patients do after such invasive surgery. Antonio was pleased that his dog had done so well, and, as agreed, he paid his fees in full with crisp, fresh bills.

I often think of Greco and Antonio. No one before or since has so clearly articulated the contract between myself, my clients, and my patients. It is indeed a sacred trust to have in my care the object of someone's love and devotion. It's a responsibility that is sometimes simple, sometimes tough, sometimes funny, but always full of emotion — hope or sadness, joy or pathos. Some patients, like Greco, recover fully and never look back. Others never improve, stubbornly immune to even our best efforts. Some diagnoses are as stunningly obvious as Greco's stone. Others are unclear and remain just beyond comprehension, straining our knowledge and experience to fit the pieces of the diagnostic puzzle together.

Throughout the meandering course of each case, though, I am aware of the bond between the patient and its person, the owner's paralyzing fear of loss, the level of trust being placed in me. And I am reminded again to "teka de responsibility to fixa de dohg."

MILK FEVER

All veterinarians can look back to their past and identify a veterinary mentor who fostered their interest in the profession, acted as an adviser and often an employer, and wrote letters of recommendation for admission committees the country over. Mine was Dr. Virgil Boyd, a mixed-animal practitioner in the small farming community of Hutchinson, Minnesota, where I attended high school. He did all of those things for me and more. I worked for him in his clinic in the mornings and attended classes in the afternoons. To this day, I owe Dr. Boyd a huge debt for the interest he invested in me and the experiences he provided.

Dr. Boyd seemed to me, at the age of seventeen, to be a man of considerable intellect, wisdom, and age. Given my age now, I recognize that he was not really very old at all. But at the time, I viewed him as nearing retirement. This misperception seems especially ironic now, since Dr. Boyd, well into his eighties, with a full head of gray hair and a regal beard of the same hue, is still a solo practitioner in Hutchinson. I visited him at his clinic last fall when I attended my thirtieth high school homecoming weekend.

Rural Minnesota is populated by a unique breed of people. Minnesotans are a hardy, self-sufficient, and thoroughly dependable people who are firmly grounded in the values of hard work, family, country, and God. Every community, regardless of size, has at least two things: a grain elevator and a thriving Lutheran church. Every self-respecting Minnesota Lutheran, as a way of life, will go out of his way to help a stranger. They do this as an outgrowth of their strong Christian values, of course. But they also do it with an ever-present knowledge that in the clutches of a cruel Minnesota winter, a person in a broken-down car will in short order become a Popsicle without the assistance of his neighbors. They are also acutely aware that their own car could break down.

Minnesota Lutherans are honest, sturdy, guileless, and strangers to coarseness. This is not to say they are prudes. The earthy conversation in most milking parlors includes descriptions of bovine waste products that in any other setting would be considered swearing. But for farmers who spend their lives shoveling the stuff, it is more professional terminology than expletive. Most devout Minnesota Lutheran farmers would sooner slice off their own leg than unleash a barrage of ear-burning curses.

Dr. Boyd was not a tall person, but he was large in every way. He was barrel-chested, with a prominent stomach. He had a huge head with a wild shock of prematurely graying hair set on top of his head like the flame of a torch, uncontrollable and waving indiscriminately; and similar to dealing with a flame, he made few attempts to constrain it. He had a large beard with streaks of gray in it that looked to be contaminating their surrounding neighbors. Even his glasses were large and dark, with huge lenses. These and his immense personality gave him an impressive presence.

Dr. Boyd was not a farmer, and he did not share a burning religious fervency. But he was a Minnesota Lutheran veterinarian serving Lutheran Minnesota farmers. Any good Lutheran knows that justification is the work of a moment. But sanctification is the work of a lifetime, and this process in Dr. Boyd was not yet complete. Though he was a churchgoing man, I had seen on occasion his penchant for emotional explosions and colorful language when things fell apart unexpectedly. Heaven knows, I had once been the recipient of a verbal volcano when I had accidentally broken the glass barrel of a syringe he needed for his next farm call. Despite these idiosyncrasies, he was adored by the farmers in the community. I looked up to him immensely.

I knew he knew this about me. And it was clear that he took his responsibilities as my mentor seriously, carefully instructing me in lessons of animal husbandry, veterinary career choices, and a life well lived. I accompanied Dr. Boyd often on his rounds in the truck, careening around the county at top speed down roads piled on each side with mountains of salt-slicked snow, like the dry ground in the Red Sea upon which the children of Israel crossed. Every large animal veterinarian I know drives the back roads like a drunken soldier on the last night of furlough. This is essential, it seems, as every farm call is considered by the farmer to be an emergency. Besides, more calls can be crammed into the span of time between sunrise and sunset when they are done at full throttle. Though I would be wise to follow Dr. Boyd's example in navigating life, I would be a fool to navigate country roads as he did.

I was not permitted to attend Dr. Boyd on his rounds until he had escorted me to the local dry-goods store and outfitted me with a pair of blue coveralls and rubber boots that fit over my shoes. The fact that the boots were rubber allowed me to scrub them carefully before leaving every farm. I doused them with a solution of warm water, which he dispensed from the tank in his Bowie veterinary box, mixed with the dark green and luminously scented disinfectant Roccal. So much a part of rural Minnesota veterinary practice was this ceremonious cleansing that every mixed-animal practice I had ever been in smelled strongly of Roccal, a pervasive medical smell with a lingering metallic odor. To my mind, it is still what the color green smells like.

Whether this habit truly prevented the spread of contagious diseases between farms or was merely a way for Dr. Boyd to impress the farmers with his thoroughness and keep the interior of his truck clean, I really don't know. But I can still picture him sitting on the tailgate of his truck, one leg thrown carelessly across his knee while sloshing the Roccal solution over his muck-covered boots with a blue-bristled brush, his head glistening with sweat and the frost from his breath circling around his head as he chuckled easily with the farmer. It was an entirely comfortable and wholesome scene.

The time I spent in Dr. Boyd's truck was invaluable for me. I had no previous cattle experience, so each trip was filled with new occurrences. I particularly remember one perfectly clear and bitterly cold day in late January. I had classes in the afternoon and was scheduled to accompany Dr. Boyd on three farm calls that morning. I had arrived early at the office, an old house situated one block off Main Street, to clear the empty glass bottles out of the truck from the previous day's calls and replenish the sundry supplies and medications. I was just pulling on my coveralls as Dr. Boyd drove in and approached the truck, carrying a steaming Thermos of hot coffee.

The first call was to a farm on the northwest end of town. I was relieved to see that the patient was standing in a thirty-by-forty-foot pen in a building that was enclosed on three sides and well protected from the northern arctic wind that blew easily through even the thickest layers of clothing. On one end of the pen, the fences narrowed to a chute with a head gate that immobilized the cows, enabling us to safely examine them. On the other end, there was an acute angle in the corner where the fences met. Our patient was a yearling Holstein heifer standing in the middle of the pen with a foot held up awkwardly, the skin around the top of the hoof red and swollen.

"Bruce," called Dr. Boyd as we approached the pen, "go on in there and chase that heifer into the chute so I can catch her head. We won't want to deal with that foot without some restraint."

It seemed unwise of me to enter that pen with the nine-hundred-pound beast, but there was no way I was going to let Dr. Boyd see my reticence. Immediately, I scaled the five-foot-high wood-rail fence and jumped down into the pen. I could feel ice forming in my veins as the great head turned to assess the scrawny person who had entered the pen with her. She was facing the open side of the building, peacefully chewing her cud, the picture of domestication. I looked questioningly at Dr. Boyd for further instructions.

"Go to the side away from the chute. She'll turn away from you and head into it. I'll clamp the chute on her neck once her head's through."

I skirted to the right side of the cow, giving her a wide berth, then positioned myself just in front of the acute angle in the corner and started in with what I thought were irresistible cattle-prodding phrases.

"Get along there, heifer," I offered weakly. The cow did not move. In fact, it lazily turned its head away from me again.

"Gonna have to say it like you mean it. And she won't move unless you do. Go ahead and move in closer." I could hear Dr. Boyd chuckle under his breath.

His mirth at my inexperience motivated me more than his encouragement. With an assertiveness born of embarrassment, I shouted at the cow and moved toward her, waving my arms. I had not moved more than a step or two when the cow did turn, but not in the direction of the chute. Before I could react, she was facing me full-on. I did not know cattle expressions well, but I was sure she was fixing me with a malevolent glare. Then two things happened simultaneously.

One was an urgent shout from Dr. Boyd. What was it he said? Something like "Get out of there NOW!" At the same time, I realized that the cow was charging me, her head down, moving at a surprising speed, given the lack of room to accelerate. Then the flat of her forehead hit me full in the chest, the force of the blow smashing me against the wooden rails in the corner where the fences met. It evacuated the air from my lungs with such force that I let out an involuntary grunt, loud and long. There were no words, just a guttural yell of primal proportions. Then the heifer turned and ran into the chute, where Dr. Boyd snapped the head gate closed around her neck.

I was completely unhurt, though surprised beyond belief. Despite the abruptness of the impact, I had been hit harder during games of flag football, although never by a player who outweighed me by a thousand pounds. Fortunately, the heifer had no horns. Only the flat expanse of her forehead had impacted my chest. The fence had kept me from flying backward and ending up feet over tail amid the manure. I was simply stunned and remained standing in the corner with my arms spread across the top rails, crosslike. The only person more surprised than I, perhaps, was Dr. Boyd, who raced to the corner where I was standing, his eyes wide and entreating.

"You okay?" he asked, breathless, no doubt visions of legal liability flooding his consciousness.

"I'm fine. Just surprised, that's all."

The rest of the farm visit fades from my memory. Dr. Boyd did something with the foot after tying it up to the rails of the chute. But I cannot recall the details. The look in that cow's eyes was too firmly imprinted on my brain to concentrate on much else.

The next call was five or six miles to the west. Dr. Boyd kept up a steady monologue while driving at breakneck speed down the snowy roads. I'm sure his purpose was to engender within me a level of continued enthusiasm for veterinary medicine. His ongoing discourse centered on the ways to best protect yourself from the sundry methods a half-ton animal has to disable you. But my mind was still abuzz with memories of the impact of that huge head.

As we drove onto the farm, Dr. Boyd was in the midst of assuring me that this call would go better and I would be in no danger. Our patient here was a cow that had recently freshened. Dr. Boyd had used this term as if I knew what it meant, which I did not. It was not until I asked for clarification that I learned it meant she had just had a calf. This particular beast had failed to pass the placenta after calving. Our task would be to remove the retained placenta. I knew these calls were designated in the appointment book simply as RPs. But I had no concept of what this entailed. We gathered the supplies and medications he thought he would need, placing them in a stainless-steel bucket, and headed into the barn.

My first sense was one of relief when I saw that the cows in the barn were lined up facing the outside walls, their heads in stanchions that kept them in place but allowed adequate room for them to move and tug at the hay that was placed in the mangers in front of them. No rodeos here, I thought.

My second sense was to wish I had one sense less. Filling the entire expanse of the barn was a powerful stench that would have made a coroner gag. To say that the barn reeked would be like saying that sugar is sweet, an offense to the definitive example of an entire genre of sensory experience. I realized that that smell could well be the measure against which all future uses of the word would forever be compared. It was the embodiment of decay; the scent equivalent of blasphemy; a putrid presence insinuating itself into my nostrils, my sinuses, my insides and filling me with a revulsion from which there was no escape. Holding my breath did not help. The smell was a living thing that appropriated my skin, burrowing into it, breaching it, and invading through it directly into my bloodstream. My eyes began to water and my nose to drip in protest. I wanted to turn and run to the relative freshness of the manure pond we had passed on the way into the barn, drinking deeply of the refreshing scents there, almost floral by comparison. But I had to follow Dr. Boyd, who was clearly ignoring the screaming voices of common sense that most beings with cognitive abilities and the power of ambulation would have heeded.

I did not think it possible for the smell to strengthen. But as we plunged deeper through the cloud of putrefaction, the smell grew larger and more intense. About the time I thought my consciousness would desert me, I saw, through the almost visible vale of odor, that Dr. Boyd was setting the stainless-steel bucket down behind a cow that was placidly pulling at the hay in front of her. She would have seemed normal had it not been for the purple-and-red trail of decaying tissue hanging from her backside. It was from this disgusting mass of rotting material that the smell was emanating.

"That is a retained placenta," Dr. Boyd said, smiling.

I couldn't conceive how he was able to smile. I could not bring myself to part my lips even to speak. I just nodded dumbly, my face squinched up in a feeble attempt to close my nostrils.

"It's awful, isn't it?"

I nodded again, thinking that I might have to deposit my breakfast into the gutter behind the cow. Gutters in dairy barns are ingenious inventions. In Minnesota, every dairy barn has the same system. The center aisle of the barn is about six feet wide. It is bordered on each side by a ten-inch-wide gutter, which is eight or ten inches deep. At the bottom of this trench is a conveyer-belt contraption that catches and transports the manure along the gutter, depositing it finally into a manure pond situated beside the barn. The manure pond is generally fifty or more feet across and perhaps four feet deep. To the contents of this pond are added water and a few other ingredients from a carefully developed recipe and mixed with the raw materials provided by the cows. Every so often, this swill is sucked up into the semi-size manure spreader and sprayed as fertilizer on the fields, a smelly job. It was a job I grew to despise when, several years after the visit described here, I worked for a summer on a dairy farm in Wisconsin. As a joke, the farmer I worked for had installed a diving board on the side of the manure pond.

"This is one of the worst jobs we have to

do in veterinary medicine. Now you can understand why we hate to get these calls." It was true. Many times I had seen his face fall when one of his clients called with this complaint. "What do you think of it?"

Finally, my speech centers recovered enough to respond. "It's hideous, horrible. What in the world happens to cause this?"

"Well, most of the time after a calf is born, the placenta is delivered in just a few minutes. But occasionally, the connections between the placenta and the uterus don't break down like they're supposed to. They hang like that for a while and the tissues start to decay. We usually get the call to come out after they've been hanging there for three or four days — just at their worst."

While he was describing the problem to me, I watched in horror as he slipped his right arm out of the sleeve of his coveralls, tucking the empty sleeve inside the waist. He then pulled on a shoulder-length plastic sleeve, working his fingers carefully down to the ends of the glove, and squeezed a generous portion of lubricant onto his now-gloved hand.

"What do you have to do to remove it?" I asked, afraid that I might find out.

"You just have to slip your hand up into the uterus and break down the connections that are holding the placenta in. I do this with my right hand and provide gentle traction on the tissue hanging out with my left. It feels kinda like separating Velcro." He worked steadily as he talked, his arm inserted into the cow up to the shoulder. Before long, he let the vile three-foot-long section of placenta fall into the gutter behind the cow. He looked pleased with himself.

"How do you prevent this from happening?"

"Well, the textbooks all say that there's nothing proven to effectively prevent retained placentas. It's just something that happens." He leaned in close and continued in a conspiratorial tone. "But I have found something that has worked in most cases to avoid these types of farm calls."

"Really? What's that?"

He looked up and down the barn, as if scouring a crowd for gunmen. The farmer had gone to retrieve some warm water for cleaning the stench from Dr. Boyd's arms. Then he turned to me again and spoke in my ear.

"I teach the farmers how to do this on their own." He held my gaze for a moment before breaking into laughter, proud of his wit.

"Now all we need is a quick shot of penicillin. Don't want this to turn into an infection. That would be awful." I handed him the huge barrel-size syringe filled with the thick white penicillin solution he had drawn up at the truck, and with a single deft motion, he expertly deposited liquid into the muscles of the cow's thigh. "That ought to do it."

He stepped back and pulled the plastic glove from his arm, turning it inside out as he did so. The farmer came back into the barn toting a bucket with steam rising above its rim. With a towel, Dr. Boyd began to rub the extraneous debris from his arms. In less time than it takes to describe it, the cow began to stiffen, her nose reaching up and forward and her tail pointing skyward. Then she began to shudder and tremble and from deep within her a bawl went out that sent shivers down my spine. Then she simply collapsed, falling onto her buckled legs as if she had been assassinated by an unseen sniper, and then she toppled onto her side. She did not breathe. She did not move. There was no spark of life in her eyes.

My reaction was to drop my jaw in astonishment. Dr. Boyd's was to take off at a dead run like a sprinter off the blocks. With unspoken questions on our lips, the farmer and I watched him push through the closed door as if it was not there. He was out of sight for only a few seconds before he was racing once more toward us, drawing medication from a dark amber bottle with a syringe as he ran. When he reached the downed cow, he plunged the needle of the syringe deep into her neck, pushing the medication into her vein as fast as he could. Then he stood up, breathing hard, and stared silently at the cow, concern on his face.

Nothing happened for three or four seconds. Then the cow began to quiver again as she had before she'd collapsed. Another bellow escaped from her. Ten seconds later, she lifted her head and looked around like a drunk coming to after a binge. She seemed almost embarrassed, as if her collapse had been an unforgivable impropriety. She heaved herself back onto her chest before rising again. Within a minute of that injection, she was once again chewing idly at her hay.

I was dumbfounded, but Dr. Boyd turned to the farmer as if this was just what he had expected and gave instructions to him about aftercare for the cow and withdrawal times for the medications he had administered. Before I knew it, we had scrubbed our boots and were driving out of the farmyard.

"What happened?" I was almost shrieking. "Why did she go down like that? And how did you get her back so quickly?"

"That is called 'anaphylactic shock.' It doesn't happen very often, but it is dramatic when it does. The cow had an allergic reaction to the penicillin. When it happened, I ran out to the truck and got some epinephrine. I knew I had to get it into her vein while her heart was still pumping, or we'd have no chance to save her. I wasn't sure if I'd made it in time till she started coming around again."

I have seen near-fatal anaphylactic allergic reactions only a few times in the twenty-three years I have been in practice. Each time, it has been as sudden, unexpected, and dramatic as the first time I witnessed it in the dead of a Minnesota winter in a dairy barn.

"That was amazing," I whispered.

"Yeah, it was, wasn't it? And something else good about it."

"What's that?" I asked.

"It made you forget about the smell, didn't it?"

"Nothing will ever make me forget that smell. Not ever! At least not until I'm as dead as that cow was."

■ ■ ■ ■

"We have one more call this morning before you have to get to class. This one is a milk fever case."

"What is milk fever? An infection in the milk?" I asked.

Dr. Boyd chuckled. "No, it has nothing to do with the milk, actually. Many of the diseases were named before we knew what caused them. The old names usually stick, though. Milk fever is a calcium deficiency that often develops around calving time, when the cows begin to produce lots of milk. The lack of calcium makes it so the muscles stop working and the cows can't walk or move. In many cases, the cows actually collapse. It can be life-threatening for both the cow and her calf, so for the farmers, it can be a double loss. At least that's what I'm expecting to find. We'll see when we get there."

The ride was enjoyed in silence, both of us breathing in the sweet fresh air from the windows we had left cracked to the icy air. I was still recovering from the olfactory onslaught, and frankly, Dr. Boyd was still pretty ripe. From the way he looked at me, I suspected he felt the same about me. As we neared our destination, he turned to address me.

"Just so you know, this farmer is a bit unique."

"Oh yeah? In what way?"

"Well, among Minnesota Lutherans, he's particularly devout. I always am careful to mind my P's and Q's when I'm on his farm. He's one of the few farmers I know who calls cow manure, manure. So watch yourself here."

"Dr. Boyd, have you ever heard me swear?"

"No, I haven't, but this is not the place to start."

Once on the farm, we loaded the ubiquitous stainless-steel bucket with supplies. Included among them were two or three of the brown glass bottles that I was accustomed to cleaning and sterilizing at the office. I had not known what their use was, and I was pleased to think I might find out. We then followed the farmer into the barn.

It was clear immediately which of the many cows in the barn was our patient. While most of them were standing in their stanchions, absentmindedly chewing on wisps of hay, one heifer was lying flat out on her side, her fanny hanging over the gutter. Her breathing was shallow and her sides

73

intermittently quivered with involuntary spasms that shuddered from her nose to her tail. She was clearly very close to calving, her huge abdomen bloated beyond belief.

Dr. Boyd knelt beside her and listened to her heart with his stethoscope while at the same time feeling the pulse in her carotid artery. The cow's eye followed him as he moved around her, though she was unable to move her neck to do so. He then turned his attention to her distended abdomen. Placing his clenched fist against her side, he pushed it deep into her belly, feeling the full-term calf bump up against it. I could see the cow's side move as the calf responded to this insult. At least the calf was still alive, even if its mother appeared too far gone to save.

Dr. Boyd positioned me at the cow's head and gave me a dose of liquid in a one-liter amber bottle to which he had attached a long section of sterile plastic tubing. I watched as he slipped a needle the size of a sixpenny nail into the cow's jugular vein. He gave me instructions to hold the bottle up at shoulder height as the fluid flowed through the tubing and into the dying cow.

"That's a calcium solution to replace this cow's calcium deficits. It usually works pretty quickly and it's almost a miracle. If it goes in too quickly, though, there can be some effects on the heart rhythm. So I'll listen for a bit while it flows. If I tell you to slow it down, hold the bottle lower; hold it higher if I tell you to speed it up."

I watched as he listened through the stethoscope to the cow's heart, directing the speed of calcium flow by positioning the height of the bottle. I was the orchestra, he the maestro. But it was a symphony only he could hear. He and the cow — who appeared to be feeling better already — I presume. Abruptly, he got up from kneeling beside the cow and began to strip the clothing from his upper body, exposing a large but powerful pearly white Minnesota chest and belly.

"Milk fever completely paralyzes the muscles in a cow. It leaves both the voluntary muscles and the involuntary muscles useless. This cow is ready to calve, but she can have no contractions with her calcium so low. This is actually helpful for me now because I can feel the position of the calf and turn it if necessary without fighting against the labor contractions. Uterine contractions can squeeze the heck out of your arm." I saw a look of horror cross his face, and he turned to the farmer.

"Pardon my French, Tom." The farmer

turned a cold, disapproving eye on him and nodded curtly.

Dr. Boyd then lubricated his right arm with a sterile lubricant and lay down on the floor behind the cow, inserting his arm up to the shoulder into her birth canal. It was an unbelievable sight for me as a junior in high school: a man with eight years of higher education stripped to the waist on the floor of a frigid Minnesota dairy barn, his body bridging the manure-filled gutter and his arm buried to the hilt inside a downed cow. The irony of it hit me as I held the calcium solution aloft.

If I still flirted with any temptations to become a dairy practitioner, that day had quashed it. This was the third in a series of career-defining calls. I resolved in my mind at that moment as I surveyed the scene before me that horse practice was my goal. What happened next, though, sealed the deal.

I could sense that as the fluid flowed into that cow's veins, her strength was returning. At first, she was just able to lift her head and gaze behind her at the man lying in the gutter. She seemed to be as surprised as I was. Then I realized that the muscles of her tail had begun to work, and she was able finally to flick it around at the annoying occurrences at her posterior. Since it had been hanging uselessly in the manure trench for many hours, this was particularly unpleasant for Dr. Boyd, who was having his chest and back painted liberally with the stuff. I was impressed with his self-control, for he avoided using a few choice words when confronted with this indignity.

From the wincing that began to be apparent on his face, I knew that the uterus was now starting to contract, inflicting viselike squeezes on his arm. Suddenly, the cow took a particularly deep breath and bore down with a mighty grunt. Unfortunately, the uterus was not the only thing that had not contracted for a long time. The cascade of fecal matter that erupted from just below the cow's tail was epic in proportion and force. Wave after wave of brown and green poured forth over Dr. Boyd's shoulder and back as he lay there. It flowed down over his ear, filling it before continuing down his cheek and caking his beard. It filled the space between his glasses and his eyes, which he squinched tightly closed. His head looked like a bust over which chocolate had been poured, like a chocolate fountain at a wedding reception.

With some effort, he extracted his arm from the cow's behind and stood, holding his breath to avoid inhaling the excreta that covered his face. First, he removed his glasses, and the dammed poo fell from his eyes to the floor. Then, using both hands, he squeegeed the poop from his face with his fingers and blew it from his nostrils with the force of a blast from a whale's blowhole. Like a wet dog, he shook his head, sending manure in all directions, flecking my coveralls with it and leaving brown spots on the whitewashed walls of the barn some eight feet away.

I could see the color building on his torso, redness creeping toward his shoulders as he leaned down and grabbed a clean towel from the stainless-steel bucket. With it, he wiped his face clean enough so that I could appreciate the redness of the mounting fury burning on his cheeks. The frustration was intense, building second by second. I could sense it in his clenched teeth and the taut lines of his lips. With concern, I realized that his pent-up vitriol would soon erupt into a cosmic outburst, and I glanced furtively at the farmer. His cheeks were trembling and I could see mirth behind the cloak of his eyes.

Vibrations began emanating from somewhere in the neighborhood of Dr. Boyd's liver. His great belly began to quiver with burgeoning anger, redder now than I could believe. A low, building groan started in his throat, his Adam's apple pumping up and down like a piston. With difficulty, he kept his lips closed to prevent the predictable verbiage from spilling out. But the effort was just too much. The groan became a grunt, and the force within the human pressure cooker was reaching critical proportions. I knew he was about to let fly with an earth-shattering barrage.

"Gggggaaa . . ." it began. Then I noticed his gaze turn to the farmer, whose face was set in a grimace born either of righteous indignation or overwhelming laughter. The distinction was not clear, but apparently at that moment, Dr. Boyd decided not to risk offending this longtime client. As the tectonic pressures finally overtook him, he let loose with the strongest oath he felt he could unleash in the presence of this devout Lutheran.

"Ggggg . . . GOLLY!"

The utter inadequacy of the expletive broke the dam of restraint in both the farmer and me, and we were rendered completely helpless by the laughter that erupted from us. We melted, weak and blathering onto our knees, roiling in bellyaching laughter. After a few seconds, I was relieved to see the lines on Dr. Boyd's face softening, and before long he, too, was helpless with mirth. The three of us laughed for quite some time. Only a long grunt from the patient and the plopping of a healthy, squirming calf at our feet finally stopped us. It was a satisfying end to a farm call, and a typical morning in dairy practice. It was also the end of any thoughts on my part of spending my life as a cow doctor.

My Day with the Horse Vets

After the debacle with Dr. Boyd and the cattle calls, he realized that cow medicine was not in my future. Squelching his disappointment, he approached me one day during my senior year in high school with a suggestion.

"Say, Bruce, I was thinking," he said. "I'm probably not going to get you pumped up for dairy practice, am I?"

"I just can't see myself spending all my time with cows," I replied.

"Your interest is in horse practice, right?"

"Yeah, horses are really my first love," I responded. "Why do you ask?"

"I have some colleagues over in Maple Plain who have a very busy and successful equine practice. I bet they would be willing to have you join them for a day to see what a horse practitioner does. Would you be interested in that?"

"Oh yeah! That would be amazing. I'd

love that!" I exclaimed.

It was several weeks before he was able to schedule my day with the horse vets, and I was impatient. Finally, the day arrived and I drove the thirty-five miles from Hutchinson to Maple Plain and located the hospital. I walked into the lobby and introduced myself to the receptionist behind the counter, who surveyed me carefully, seeming strangely confused.

"The doctors are in rounds in the back room," she said, nodding her head in the direction of the doors behind her. "Go on back. They're expecting you."

With eager anticipation, I made my way to the back, where I found four men in blue coveralls sitting in a darkened room and staring intently at the X-rays of a horse's foot on the view box. I could make out the unmistakable outline of the hoof surrounding an array of unfamiliar bones standing out in stark contrast to the darkness on the rest of the film. My entrance distracted them and they turned in unison and stared at me, seeming, if not annoyed, at least a bit surprised. None of them spoke.

"Hello," I said tentatively. "I'm Bruce."

Still they stared at me silently, taking me in from my head to my leather boots. I was arrayed, as they were, in the blue coveralls that Dr. Boyd had purchased for me to go on farm calls. I thought I looked like quite the professional.

"Dr. Boyd worked it out for me to ride with one of you guys?"

"Oh yeah, now I remember," the oldest of the men said, breaking into a smile and offering his hand for a firm shake. "I'm Dr. Evers, the senior partner in this practice. And this is Dr. Conner, Dr. Vick, and Dr. Carroll."

I shook each man's hand as he was introduced to me, honored beyond measure at their apparent pleasure to meet me. The pleasure, though, was all mine.

"Virgil said you are interested in horse practice," Dr. Evers said. "Is that right?"

"Yes, sir, I am. I've wanted to be an equine vet for as long as I can remember."

This seemed to resonate with the group. I was enormously impressed by the four professionals in the room, who were doing exactly what I envisioned myself doing one day. But that was still a long way off. A minimum of eight and a half years of additional schooling stretched interminably ahead of me before I would be qualified to sit in their seats. They turned back to the case they were discussing but took the time to bring me up to speed on the details.

"This is a five-year-old Thoroughbred gelding that has a non-weight-bearing lameness on the right front," Dr. Evers said, recapping. He was obviously the attending clinician on this case. "This horse belongs to a woman who does dressage with him. He's her best hope for the show circuit this season, so she's pretty motivated to get this problem taken care of."

"I see," I responded with as much confidence as I could muster, surrounded as I was by men whom I so admired.

"What year are you in school, Bruce?"

"I'm a senior," I replied proudly. "I graduate this year!"

Dr. Evers nodded his head and turned again to the X-rays. The room quieted and I could sense that a change had set in among the men.

"So take a look at the X-rays and tell me what's causing the lameness in this horse."

I felt my face begin to redden in the darkness. I wanted so badly to impress them with my prodigious horse knowledge, gained from years of reading outdated issues of *Western Horseman* magazine and my two summers as a camp wrangler. But nothing so far had prepared me for this grilling by four seasoned medical professionals.

"I don't know," I said flatly, embarrassed

by my ignorance. I saw a wave of disbelief wash over the group. Looks of helplessness flashed on their faces as they exchanged glances. Dr. Evers raised his eyebrows and sighed heavily before continuing the questioning.

"We don't mean to put you on the spot. But can you come up with a list of differentials for a non-weight-bearing lameness in a five-year-old horse?" The room went silent again. I could hear the ticking of the clock on the wall. The four men waited for my response.

"Well, I guess he could have a broken leg," I offered weakly. The silence in the room was in stark contrast to the ringing in my ears. I was glad the lights were low, so they would not see the blushing of my face deepen.

"Anything else?"

"Maybe an abscess?" I added hesitantly. Dr. Evers nodded sternly. I continued: "Or he might have foundered. Or maybe there's a nail or something that punctured the sole."

"Do you see a nail on the X-ray?"

I surveyed the film carefully, then shrugged. "I don't know."

One of the other doctors took over the interrogation at that point — kind of a good cop/bad cop thing, it seemed. I think it was

Dr. Conner, though their names were already fading from my mind under the glare of their mounting displeasure. With an edge of frustration to his voice, he turned to me.

"There's no nail on the film, Bruce. Clearly this is a case of laminitis. You can tell it by the rotation of the coffin bone here away from the edge of the hoof wall. Can you see that?"

"Oh yeah. That's pretty cool." I chuckled appreciatively. I had never seen an X-ray of a horse's foot before and I found it amazingly exhilarating, despite the fact that these men were clearly becoming increasingly put out with me.

"So what would you do for a case of laminitis this severe?"

"I guess I'd call you guys," I said, laughing at my ready wit, but slightly concerned when none of them laughed, too. There was another moment of awkward silence before Dr. Evers abruptly stood up.

"Okay, so it seems we're done here. We'd better hit the road. We've got a busy day. I guess I'll take Bruce with me, unless one of you wants him." There were no takers.

I followed Dr. Evers to his truck, its gleaming white veterinary box filling the bed. We climbed in and set off on an adventure I had been looking forward to for many weeks. Our first call was to a breeding farm, where we were to perform an artificial insemination on a mare worth many thousands of dollars. The sire was a famous stallion who commanded a stud fee of $75,000. Both horses were on-site at the farm for the breeding and were to be evaluated beforehand by Dr. Evers.

"If both horses are at the farm, why not just let them breed naturally?" I asked.

"Because they are both too valuable to risk injury. It's as simple as that."

"Will you need my help, or should I just watch?"

"You can help. First, we're going to collect the stallion. Then we'll evaluate for abnormalities under a microscope before infusing it in the uterus."

None of this made a bit of sense to me. Why in the world would we collect the stallion? Hadn't he just told me he was right here at the farm? And how would he evaluate the huge horse under a microscope? All will come clear, I thought. I was here to learn from the professionals, after all.

"What do you want me to do?"

"I'll show you when the time comes. Just remember, though, you have to be quick. Things happen pretty fast in the heat of the moment."

Once on the farm, Dr. Evers removed from his truck a three-foot-long plastic two-layered sleeve reminiscent of the arm of a thick down jacket. He filled the space where the feathers would have been with warm water. This left a hollow tubelike space between these water-filled layers. He lubricated this space generously with a slippery goo he squeezed from a tube. He attached an eight-inch-long plastic funnel to one end of this contraption, and to that he affixed a large test tube.

"What in the world is that thing?" I asked.

"That thing is what you are going to hand me when I ask for it. It is the most important piece of equipment in this whole process. Handle it carefully," he said, placing it gingerly in my arms.

The mare was brought into the aisle of the barn and cross-tied with a rope from each side. Dr. Evers carefully examined her, starting at the head but spending most of his time at the other end. His exam included inserting his arm up to the shoulder in one orifice or another — I wasn't sure which. Apparently, she passed with flying colors because she was soon escorted back to her stall by a groom.

The stallion was then brought out by another stable hand and led to an arena with a circumference of some one hundred feet. It was not clear who was in control of whom, but the groom seemed to have the upper hand, with the help of a leather lead with a two-foot length of brass chain at its end, which was snapped to one side of the halter, looped over the horse's nose, and passed through the D-ring on the groom's side of the stallion. Every step or two, the groom would give the lead a quick jerk. This reminded the powerful beast to follow directions despite the surging of his raging hormones. As an experienced stud horse, he knew exactly what his immediate future held.

Dr. Evers carefully examined the stallion as well, concentrating his efforts on the animal's reproductive apparatus. When he was satisfied that all was in order, he directed the workers to bring the mare into the arena and then positioned me to one side. In my arms I held the odd paraphernalia he had assembled. The effect of the receptive mare on the amorous stallion was akin to adding jet fuel to a Boy Scout's campfire. He began to dance and whinny, his neck flexed so tightly that his chin nearly brushed his chest, sweat quickly springing to his neck and sides. It was only with the greatest of difficulty that the frantic groom could maintain any control at all on the glistening horse as he approached the mare.

When it was clear that the stallion was about to commence operations, Dr. Evers called me close and took from me the six-pound water balloon. With one hand, he grabbed the stallion's thrusting equipment and diverted it into the lubricated plastic tube he held in the other. That's what that thing is for! There was intense activity for a few seconds, some loud grunting, and then the stallion was backing away. It was perhaps the most intense, frenetic, and injury-prone event I had ever witnessed. If these two horses were too valuable to risk injury doing a natural breeding, it made me wonder about the value of the veterinarian who had clearly risked life and limb to achieve an artificial one.

Dr. Evers turned on his heels, cradling the contraption carefully in his arms like a newborn. The test tube was now full of a very valuable thick fluid, which he took to a table on which he had set up a makeshift laboratory with a microscope, several test tubes, slides, and papers. For a few minutes, he looked carefully through the microscope's eyepieces, evaluating the shape, number, and motility of the great horse's sperm. He even let me look through the microscope at the millions of squirming tadpoles while he made some notes on a pad of paper.

He then sucked up the fluid in a syringe, which he attached to a three-foot-long thin plastic pipette. Guiding the advancement of this tube into the mare's uterus with a gloved arm inserted into her, he had me infuse the entire aliquot of semen through the tube, depositing it just where it needed to be. It was a thrilling drama for me to play even the smallest of parts in.

In the truck again, Dr. Evers turned to me. "Any questions?"

Any questions? I was brimming with them. Everything that had just happened was completely new to me. Why let the stud mount the female at all if you were trying to minimize the risk of injury? What were you looking for when you studied the sperm under the microscope? How long did the sample remain viable? How were you able to find the right place to deposit the sample in the mare? But my mind froze. I simply could not organize my questions into a logical sequence. And when I opened my mouth, the question that actually came out was one I had not even considered.

"How could you tell when the stallion was . . . you know . . . done?"

Dr. Evers's head sank in apparent disbelief tainted with what seemed like disappointment and he shook it slowly. "You just know," he said quietly. "You just know."

The next job was to geld a young horse on the same farm. We drove the quarter mile to the next barn on a tree-lined lane between beautifully groomed paddocks outlined by gleaming white four-rail fences. We pulled up in the stone-paved semicircular driveway and stopped under the heavy beams that supported the overhang by the front door of the barn's stone facade.

Carrying the necessary equipment down the wide aisle of the barn, whose stall doors bore brass nameplates announcing the four-word names of the horses within, a realization dawned on me. The gulf between these horses and the somnolent animals I was used to dealing with at camp, and between this rarefied air and the camp's pole barn constructed with roughhewn creosoted two-by-sixes, was akin to the space between South Central L.A. and Buckingham Palace. I knew nothing of the world these skilled practitioners inhabited every day. It was a humbling epiphany, and intimidating.

In a ring at one end of the barn, several attendants were gathered around an impressive yearling colt, who eyed us apprehensively and circled his groom at the end of a rope. This, I knew, was our patient: a sixteen-hand bay stallion with four white socks and a wide blaze on his nose. He was in beautiful flesh and his coat gleamed with the sheen of perfect health and ideal nutrition.

Dr. Evers laid out several thick ropes and a clean towel, on which he placed some carefully wrapped packs that had been recently autoclaved. He deftly slapped a large-bore needle into the jugular vein of the horse and quickly infused a syringeful of a clear fluid into the vein. Within a couple of minutes, the horse's anxiety eased and he stood still, his great head sagging. Dr. Evers used the ropes to weave an intricate web around the colt's legs in just the perfect pattern that a gentle tug on one end tipped him onto his side and prevented him from regaining his feet. Another injection into the bulging vein and the horse went still on the ground, though his eyes remained disarmingly open.

As if on cue, the attendants began scrubbing the horse's scrotum and testicles for the surgery. Clearly, they had assisted Dr. Evers with this procedure many times. Dr. Evers opened the packs he had laid on the towel, donned a pair of sterile surgical gloves, and instructed me to do the same. He pulled a scalpel handle out of the pack and attached to it a sharp new surgical blade. Without hesitation, he knelt beside the downed horse and grasped one of the baseball-size organs in his hand. With a quick flick of his wrist, he sliced through the skin and in short order was holding the testicle, which was still tethered to the horse by a thick cord of tissue. He turned to me.

"Can you hand me the emasculator? But be sure to touch nothing but the handles."

It sounded to me like an instrument of torture, which I guess it was. I had no idea what an emasculator was or what one might look like. I turned to the open packs lying on the towel, looking for something with handles. Everything in the pack seemed to have them, so I reached for a large tool that looked like a pair of pliers and handed it to him, being careful to touch only the finger holes.

"No, that's a hemostat. I need the emasculator."

Oh, I thought. He must need something to cut with. I turned back to the open pack and reached for a huge fourteen-inch-long pair of curved scissors. These I extended to him, again being careful to touch only the finger holes.

"No, those are the Metzenbaums. Give me the emasculator. Don't you know what an emasculator is?" Dr. Evers seemed perturbed.

Wasn't it obvious that I didn't know what an emasculator was? I thought. I looked down at him with confusion on my face. He shook his head and nodded to one of the grooms, who pointed to a huge two-handled hunk of shining stainless steel that looked to me like a pair of glorified vise grips. This mean, two-fisted piece of surgical chicanery was so heavy, it almost took two hands to give it to Dr. Evers.

He took it and placed its blades around the inch-thick band of blood vessels and tissues from which hung the testicle. Checking its placement carefully, he then closed its jaws. The testicle dropped to the ground at his feet and the sleeping horse twitched his front legs involuntarily, but still Dr. Evers held the instrument with both hands, keeping it tightly clamped around the bloody stalk. He held it that way for about five minutes before tentatively loosening his grip.

He stood and turned to me with great fanfare, holding up the instrument, which now had blood dripping from its teeth like a predator, and kicked the testicle toward me with the toe of his boot. "Now that is an emasculator!" he said triumphantly. Who was I to argue? The sleeping horse was not the only one who had just been emasculated.

The opposite testicle was dispatched just as quickly and soon we were back in the truck and pulling away from the immaculate farm.

"Do they use a different kind of emasculator at the school nowadays? You didn't seem to recognize this brand."

It was true that the strict boarding school I attended was known for ironfisted enforcement of the rules, but I searched my memory for anything used at my high school that might approximate the surgical detonator I had just seen. "I don't think they even have one at my school," I replied. Out of the corner of my eye, I saw Dr. Evers cast a questioning look across the seat at me. I avoided his gaze.

"One last call before lunch," said my mentor after an awkward pause. "This is just a little laceration on the fetlock of a horse. Shouldn't take long at all. This horse man is on the other end of the spectrum from the one at the place we just left. He's a real down-to-earth guy. I think you'll like him."

After a few turns, we pulled into the long

driveway of a farm with warped, unpainted boards on the fence. The doors hung askew from their hinges and the tops of the stalls had been worn away by a long history of habitual cribbers. Cribbing is a vice that sometimes develops in bored horses that are stalled for long periods of time. They grab the boards at the top of the stall with their teeth and pull, tugging great gasps of air into their stomachs as they do so. Over time, this causes telltale damage to the wood. The taste of creosote will sometimes break this habit, so I was not surprised to see the wood at the tops of the stalls slathered with the strong-smelling tarry substance.

A middle-aged man wearing jeans and steel-toed cowboy boots came out of the barn and welcomed us with a broad smile. With a calloused hand, he swiped a stray strand of dusty hair back over the top of his rapidly balding head.

"Hello, Doug. Mighty fine day we got going, isn't it?" Dr. Evers greeted him warmly.

"Good to see you again, Dr. Evers. Who is this you got with you?"

"This is Bruce. He's going to be an equine practitioner soon and wanted to ride along with us for a day."

"You all looking to hire another doctor for

your practice, then? Already got a passel of them, don't you?"

Dr. Evers cast a furtive glance my way before answering. "No, we aren't planning on hiring Bruce here. Just hosting him for a day of observation."

"Well, it's good to meet you anyway, Bruce," Doug said. "Can't learn from any better horse doctor than Dr. Evers, that's for doggone sure. The horse I called you for is back here in the barn. He's got a right nasty little cut, too. Wouldn't have called you if I thought I could handle it myself."

We followed Doug to a stall at the far end of the barn that housed a small palomino gelding who held his right rear foot gingerly up off the ground. From a circumferential wound on his leg just below his fetlock joint, there oozed a reddish liquid, which attracted a host of flies. A pinkish mass of raw tissue bubbled out of the wound. Dr. Evers took one look at it and turned to me.

"What do you call that, Bruce?"

Finally, an answer I knew. I had spent hours in my younger years poring over anatomical diagrams of horses with arrows pointing to all the salient areas with the proper anatomical terms labeled out to the side. I had this one nailed.

"That's the fetlock joint, sir," I responded

98

proudly.

"No, not the joint, son. What do you call that gangly red tissue below the fetlock?"

I was crestfallen. I couldn't remember the last time I had been asked a question I could answer. I offered the only answer I could come up with but held no illusions that it was right.

"A scar?" I offered haltingly. I heard Doug choke back a laugh, but I didn't dare look in his direction.

"No, Bruce. Amazingly, the medical term for that tissue is not a scar." At this, Doug could contain himself no longer and he began to laugh right out loud. To my horror, Dr. Evers joined him.

"Bruce," offered Doug when his laughter died down, "that's called proud flesh."

"*Proud flesh* is the medical term for that?" I asked incredulously.

"Well, the technical name is actually exuberant granulation tissue," Dr. Evers said. "But the common name is proud flesh. For reasons we don't entirely understand, horses produce way more scar tissue than is necessary to heal a wound. And it can be very difficult to get rid of. I'm not sure why the old-timers called it proud flesh, but the name has stuck. You'll get used to it."

Dr. Evers went to work doing some type

of surgical debulking of the excessive tissue; but honestly, my heart wasn't much into it. I was distracted by a two-week-old foal in the adjacent pasture that was kicking up his heels. A sudden question from Dr. Evers brought me back to the task at hand.

"So, Bruce, after I finish cleaning this wound up, what important shot should I give this horse to make sure it doesn't get sick?"

"I guess an antibiotic injection?"

"Don't guess, man — know!" He fairly shouted the words at me. "Soon your clients will be paying you for your training and knowledge. They deserve better than your best guess. Yes, I will give him an antibiotic injection, but what preventive shot does a wound like this need?"

Though I was beyond mortified at this heated chastisement, I had no idea what Dr. Evers was referring to. I looked at him blankly but did not speak.

"My goodness, Bruce, think, for heaven's sake. It's something *you* need to get every ten years or so."

"Maybe a tetanus shot?" It was a blind stab in the dark.

"Yes, a tetanus shot! Surely you know how susceptible horses are to tetanus. Whenever they receive a penetrating injury like this, they have to have a tetanus booster. Bank on it."

"I'll remember it, sir," I said quietly. When Dr. Evers looked at me with disbelief on his face, I repeated my promise, this time defensively. "I will."

And I have remembered it ever since. If tomorrow, by some strange twist of fate, I was called out to treat proud flesh on a horse's leg, I would have not the slightest idea what the currently accepted treatment for it is. But I would, without hesitation, give the horse a tetanus shot.

I was quiet when we got back in the truck. It was only lunchtime, but already the day seemed very long — very long indeed. From the moment I had stepped foot in Dr. Evers's practice I had been grilled and interrogated for answers I did not know. Repeatedly, I had exposed my ignorance to the men whom I so wanted to impress. Nothing had gone right. I was tired and embarrassed and tired of being embarrassed. So I just sat silently in the passenger's seat, sulking. If Dr. Evers sensed my frustration, he didn't let on. And he couldn't leave well enough alone.

"Honestly, Bruce," he began after a prolonged silence. "I have some real concerns about your readiness for practice."

"I know I've got a lot to learn, but I've still got plenty of time before vet school's over."

"But graduation is only a few months away, right?"

"Yes, sir. I'm really looking forward to graduation."

"Have you gotten good grades in school?"

"Yes, sir, I have," I responded defensively. "I expect to end this semester having gotten straight A's through my whole four years."

"You're kidding me, right?" Dr. Evers seemed unimpressed by my grades.

"No, sir, I'm not. I've worked really hard for my grades." He did not respond to this for a moment, and I hoped the grilling was over. It was not.

"Do you have plans yet — after graduation, I mean?"

"Yes, sir," I responded. "I'll be working at camp this summer again. Then I'm headed to Tennessee for college."

Dr. Evers didn't really seem to be paying much attention to me, but at this comment I saw his face jerk toward me and he fixed me with a questioning look, which made me feel all the worse.

"Wait, what did you say?"

"I said I am planning to attend college in Tennessee. It's the college that both of my

brothers attended. I'm really looking forward to it."

To my utter surprise, Dr. Evers broke into
a peal of laughter that went on so long, I
began to get angry at him. He had belittled
me, bemused me, and berated me all morning long. My intelligence had been ques-
tioned, my knowledge demeaned, my future
derided. Why, even the receptionist at the
clinic had looked at me askew. I was frankly
sick of it! And here was this man, whom I
admired beyond words, laughing at me yet
again. I was about in tears when he turned
to me.

"Bruce, we owe you one great big apology, all of us!" And he went into another
prolonged round of laughter. When he had
gotten himself under control, he wiped the
streaming tears from his eyes and looked at
me with more warmth and compassion than
I had felt all day.

"When you said you were a senior this
morning at rounds, we all thought you were
a senior in veterinary school. We had no clue
that you were about to graduate from high
school. Wow, with that piece of vital information, I have to say that you have handled
yourself amazingly well. No wonder you
didn't know the answers to even the simplest
of questions. O my stars, I can't wait to tell

everyone at the office. You know, the only one who was even close was the receptionist. She said you looked awfully young."

Immediately, I felt a heavy weight roll from my shoulders. Together, we rehashed the morning's events through the eyes of each other's incorrect assumptions. Things got funnier and funnier, till we were both laughing helplessly. Needless to say, the afternoon was considerably more enjoyable than the morning had been.

As I think back on my day with the horse doctors, I still chuckle at the comedy of errors that played out at my expense. At this point in my career, I may be surprised that I do not practice equine medicine. But I doubt that Dr. Evers and his colleagues at the Maple Plain Equine Services practice are surprised one little bit.

LISA

I first met Lisa Spalding when she responded to our ad for a kennel attendant. There was nothing extraordinary about her. She had nondescript brown hair pulled into a tight ponytail. Her face was long in both dimension and demeanor, with puffy, sad eyes and buckteeth. She was lean, but not because she was in especially good physical condition. Her movements were fluid in a rather careless, almost exasperated way. The fingernails of her thumb and index finger, I noticed as I shook her hand, were nicotine-stained. I judged her to be in her late twenties, though her hardened face hinted at many more years. There was about her a veneer of self-protective nonchalance, a carefully applied indifference, as if she didn't really care whether or not she got the job. But around the edges, the veneer was a little loose, and below it I sensed an eagerness that pressed unwillingly to the surface.

True, the job for which she was applying was not very exciting: walking dogs, cleaning cages, refreshing litter boxes, a little sweeping and mopping. But I detected a spark of enthusiasm behind her mask of studied detachment. Lisa really wanted this job.

It is just this desire that I seek in applicants for openings at my hospital still — the yearning that pivots around the essence of what it is that makes a good employee in a veterinary hospital. Let's face it, it is not the fantastic pay scale that attracts people to the field. Nor is it the glamour. There's very little of that. It certainly is not the pristine work environment. Rather, it is the intangible but far more fulfilling currency of earning the trust and confidence of unruly, hurting, and confused patients and bringing them relief from their pain and discomfort. It is the compensation of seeing the tense face of a worried owner melt into joy when reunited with her healthy, tail-wagging dog or purring kitty. It is the knowledge that without your participation, this reunion would not have occurred. The kitty would not be purring and head-butting its owner; the wagging tail would be still.

Having had previous experience working in a veterinary hospital in northern Virginia,

Lisa had already cashed those emotional checks. And I could tell she wanted *this* job. She was also willing to start out doing the most menial of tasks associated with animal care. Best of all, she was willing to take the hourly wage I was able to pay her. Still, it was not without some reservations that I hired Lisa. She seemed unsettled somehow, with a dissatisfied and pessimistic approach to life. This dour outlook concerned me as I envisioned her dealing with my clients and staff. What influence would her attitude have on the interplay of the group? I well knew the negative impact one cynical, sour person could have. Lisa also seemed insecure in her mannerisms and interactions. I had worked with people in the past whose lack of self-esteem had made it difficult for them to assimilate into the mechanisms of a group. Would Lisa be able to make herself part of this team? It was a risk, but one I judged worth taking.

For the first two or three weeks, Lisa came to work and performed her duties with efficiency, but she entertained very little interaction with us. She was quiet, unsure, and tentative when we attempted to draw her out. But it was clear from the start that she had a unique ability to connect with the animals. They adored her. Even the timid, fear-biting ones responded to her quiet influence — those who hovered near the back of the kennel with heads low and tails tucked. Never afraid of even the most aggressive patients, Lisa rapidly became the go-to person for handling the few truly difficult patients that came in. As time went on, her icy persona began to thaw and we began to learn a little about her background.

She had a veritable menagerie of animals at her house, including two Border collies, which were her constant companions. Tillie, the alpha dog of her crew, had a very white face with piebald, soulful, and intelligent eyes. A few large patches of black, like island continents, floated on a sea of white fur. Unlike that of most dogs, Tillie's tail, black and full, was not a harbinger of her emotions. She kept it still and straight behind her, a rudder in the serious waters she navigated.

Life for Border collies is not what it is for Labradors, who are given to cavorting constantly in a state of never-ending celebration. Border collies are born and bred for work, with work in mind at all times. If they are not given a job of significance, they will often create one for themselves, which they will perform with unswerving devotion and dedicated attention. Such is the life of the typical Border collie.

But Tillie was not a typical Border collie. She was a Border collie on steroids, with a work ethic that made Mother Teresa seem like a slacker. And her job was to follow Lisa's every command. Her intense eyes never left Lisa's face, searching earnestly for what Lisa might want from her, often sensing even before Lisa spoke that she might want her to sit or come or lie down. Even a nod or a change of Lisa's facial expression spoke volumes to Tillie, who would respond immediately to the most subtle of cues.

Grizzly was Tillie's pup. And though he was two or three years old when I first met him, he remained an irresponsible, insolent adolescent compared to her. Grizzly was mostly dark, with hints of blue merle around his neck and in the blue iris of his left eye. You could look at Grizzly and know from his expressions and mannerisms that he had probably been up to trouble recently, but, like a scheming schoolboy, he was hard to pin down. One minute he would be haughty and glinty-eyed with mischief. The next, he would be ingratiating and compliant, desperately seeking your approval. Grizzly soon associated me with needles and unwelcome probing of some orifice or other, and he quickly developed the odd and humorous habit of squatting submissively and wetting the floor whenever I was around. Just the sound of me calling his name invariably evoked a squat, eyes suspicious and frightened, the splatter of urine hitting the floor, and a little yellow puddle pooling around his feet.

There were other animals, too. Fizz was one, the big yellow cat with a good eye and a missing one who terrorized the feline population on the dirt road where Lisa's house was situated along one of the seven bends of the Shenandoah River. There was Chewy, the affenpinscher who looked like Chewbacca from *Star Wars* and whom Lisa claimed to despise. Chewy belonged to Lisa's mother, another squatter on the property, though it was never clear to me who was the real owner and who the squatter. I even stitched a laceration once on the nose of Lisa's pygmy goat, who had flopping, dangling ears and a mouth that seemed always to be smirking at some inappropriate joke. On the flat behind the house down by the river, Lisa kept her horses, which she rarely rode, mostly because the mare, Destiny, though thoroughly broken, was hopelessly spoiled and refused to behave under a saddle.

But, though this list of Lisa's pets is not

close to complete, it was only Tillie and Grizzly who accompanied Lisa around town in her Jeep Wrangler, the canvas sides smeared with doggy slobber and the windows steamed with the excited panting of the pair. Lisa seemed most like herself while on an adventure in the Wrangler with her two dogs.

Lisa kept the intimate details of her personal story close for quite a while. But with time, we learned that she had been the teenage bride in a shotgun wedding to her high school sweetheart, Steve. The two youngsters were soon raising two youngsters of their own, Melanie and a little boy named after his father. The realities of parenthood at such an early age had pushed Steve into a workingman's trade as a painter and general handyman and sequestered Lisa within the confines of her mother's home, tending to the needs of two infants before she was twenty, the ambitious plans of her childhood fading fast, the dreams flitting like an elusive butterfly further and further from her grasp. Neither Steve nor Lisa had been able to finish high school, though Lisa later completed a GED at home between diaper changes.

After the kids got a little older, Lisa landed a part-time job at a veterinary hospital. It was there that she began to reconnect with her dreams. However, as the sprawl of Washington, D.C., seeped ever westward and escalated the cost of living in northern Virginia, Lisa's mother sought refuge by relocating her extended family to the valley. With Lisa's access to her job cut off, her world compacted again, her passion for animals sated only by her own menagerie. For Lisa, dreams deferred had become dreams denied, and each day her hopes and ambitions deflated a little more, like a progressively sagging helium balloon.

It was in one of these low ebbs that Lisa answered my advertisement and was welcomed as the newest member of my staff. Given the harsh realities of her life, I suppose it was no surprise that Lisa's outlook on life was so bleak. And yet, as time went on, I noted with pleasure that Lisa's face began to reflect a little bit of lightness, her smile coming more quickly. She displayed a sardonic, self-deprecating wit and she involved herself with the group more.

In no time at all, Lisa's skills with the patients were in demand. She learned to restrain patients as I gave injections or drew blood for laboratory testing. She became adept at reading stool samples, peering through the double eyepieces of the microscope and identifying the eggs of intestinal parasites by their unique shape and texture. She mastered the art of cowing the most rancorous of cats, bundling them into little kitty burritos with a double layer of towels as they hissed and swore, their fishy feline breath hot and angry, their sharp and swiping claws safely secured. As her responsibilities grew, so did her confidence, and a new Lisa emerged.

For some people, life tolerates no advantage. Each step forward is accompanied by a new tremor of emotion, an unexpected and undeserved new kick in the gut. Lisa was one of these people. For her, the next kick came with a nonchalant pass of her hand over Tillie's neck. She had not noticed it before, but suddenly the lymph nodes stood out under Tillie's chin like twin plums, and Tillie's usually robust appetite flagged. I happened to be on vacation when these signs were first noticed, so Lisa brought Tillie in for my associate to evaluate. She found matching growths sprouting not only under Tillie's chin but also in front of her shoulders, under her arms, and behind her knees. She had sucked a few cells from these growths with a syringe and evaluated them under the microscope and had judged them to be enflamed lymph nodes. Since she did not deem the cells to be cancerous, she had placed Tillie on a course of high-powered antibiotics to counter the effects of a suspected bacterial infection.

When I returned from vacation, Lisa told me about Tillie's illness, ending her description with the good news that the aspirate of the lymph nodes had been cancer-free and the antibiotics were expected to do the trick. A little shiver of concern started at the base of my skull and sent tendrils down my spine.

"So, how long has she been on the antibiotics?" I asked, trying to conceal my concern.

"About five days now."

"Is she any better?"

"Not yet. But I keep watching for her appetite to come back. She hasn't eaten for so long that I think she's starting to lose weight."

"Why don't you bring her in tomorrow for me to look at, just in case." I was concerned to hear that she had shown no response to the antibiotics. Usually, bacterial diseases begin to respond to appropriate antibiotic therapy within two or three days. Failure to do so means that we have either chosen the wrong antibiotic or made the wrong diagnosis.

I watched as Tillie dragged into the office the next morning, her demeanor and appearance unlike the Tillie I knew. Her eyes were not fixated on Lisa; her tail was drooping and languid. With foreboding, I ran my fingers along her neck and felt the plumpness of the lymph nodes, which usually disappear among the tissues of the body. Even in places where the nodes are usually not discernible, they stood out prominently, bulging the skin. My heart was in my throat as I plunged a needle into first one, then another of the firm, easily isolated nodules that I had trapped between my fingers.

After spraying the material from the syringes onto microscope slides, I first fixed them by holding them over the flame of a cigarette lighter, then stained them by dipping them into a series of blue, red, and purple dyes. Finally, I placed the slide under the microscope and focused down on the pink and purple cells.

Though I was not pleased to see what came into focus on the slides, I was not surprised. From one end of the slide to the other was a monotonous population of large cells, their nuclei prominent and displaying a coarse pattern of internal structure. Each nucleus hosted a number of large, bizarrely shaped structures, called nucleoli, scattered liberally throughout. There were also many cells whose nuclei were clearly in the chaotic throes of cell division, unchecked and unmitigated mitosis. All of these findings were ominous, unmistakably indicative of unrestrained growth, the hallmarks of malignancy. Tillie had cancer!

I looked through the microscope much longer than was necessary for me to make a diagnosis. I knew the telltale landmarks of lymphoma immediately. The rest of my time peering through the eyepieces was occupied in frantic rehearsal of the upcoming conversation with Lisa, which I did not relish. In her heart, though, Lisa already knew the bad news. She had suspected as much herself by the way Tillie's energy had waned and her body contours had melted away, her nodes swelling and bloating more each day.

I turned to her. My eyes, filling with concern and sympathy, met hers, which were already full of knowing and sadness. "It's not good, Lisa."

"I knew it. I just knew it!"

"This is lymphoma. And it looks like an angry case of it."

"So what does this mean?"

"Well, the prognosis is not good. Without treatment, Tillie probably has only about six or eight weeks. The good news, if there can be any good news with a diagnosis of cancer, is that lymphoma is one of the most treatable forms of cancer. In most cases, chemotherapy drugs will result in remission."

I watched Lisa's face for the familiar reaction of dismay at the mention of chemotherapy. Every client has known someone who has undergone chemotherapy for the treatment of one form of cancer or another. Everyone, it seems, reacts with some degree of repugnance to their memories of how awful the treatment regimen had been for their loved one — the racking illness that the poison of the drugs had caused, the nausea and vomiting, the draining weakness, the dehydrating diarrhea, the clumping handfuls of balding hair loss. Few clients can conceive of, or condone, their pet going through the same horrors. So it was not a surprise to see Lisa's face cloud with furrows of emotion.

"It's not what you think. Our patients don't usually get hit as hard with chemo drugs as people do. Our goal is to maintain quality of life even while we work to lengthen it. Most dogs tolerate treatment really well. And with treatment, while we don't generally achieve a cure, we can usually extend good quality of life for eight to twelve months or longer."

"It's wicked expensive, though, isn't it?" I knew this was a factor for Lisa's family. It is for most clients. It's a fair and valid consideration, too. But I also knew that Lisa would sacrifice everything for Tillie's benefit. It wouldn't be easy, but it would be easier than doing nothing, easier than watching Tillie sink into the inevitable mire of illness, waning painfully to an unavoidable end.

We started Tillie's first round of chemotherapy three days later, administering a cocktail of venomous liquid into her bloodstream, where it would target the rapidly dividing cells of the cancerous tissue. This was followed by a chaser of oral medications, which were given for four consecutive days. The next week, blood work was done to monitor the number of white blood cells. These innocent bystanders often suffer collateral damage from chemotherapy drugs and their absence can leave a patient unprotected from invading germs. Since the white-cell count was adequate, the whole process was started again. This became a weekly cycle.

Tillie tolerated the barrage of noxious toxins very well. Within a week, the size of the lymph nodes had shrunk to almost normal. This was accompanied by a marked improvement in her appetite and general well-being. At the first recheck a week later, Lisa was vastly more optimistic and had begun to see the old Tillie reemerge. By the third week, her cancer was in remission and her lymph nodes and blood work were normal. She was gaining weight, and except for a day or two after each treatment, she was back to acting like her normal self.

After a six-week induction period, Tillie's chemotherapy sessions were reduced to every three weeks, a schedule that we planned to maintain indefinitely. With the exception of a bit of barely noticeable thinning of her coat, Tillie was the picture of health for about ten months. Then Lisa once again noticed that her lymph nodes were beginning to swell. She brought Tillie back to me. I could tell by the look on Lisa's face that the situation was not good.

"Her nodes are up again. And her appetite has begun to drop off, too." Lisa reported the changes to me with calm resignation. We had known all along that this time would most likely come. When it did, we were not surprised.

I examined Tillie from nose to tail. There was no doubt about the diagnosis. Lymphoma is an awful diagnosis when first made, but resurgent chemotherapy-resistant lymphoma is worse by far. Achieving the second remission is more difficult by several orders of magnitude than winning the first round. Rescue protocols are well described in the veterinary literature, but success rates with these are lower, and disease-free intervals are much shorter than with first remissions. I knew Lisa was aware of these realities both from her own research and from experience with other cancer patients.

"Do you want to pursue further chemo for Tillie?" I asked.

"The second course would be a lot harder on Tillie, wouldn't it?"

I nodded my head.

"And second remissions don't last as long, do they?"

"You're right on both counts."

"I don't think we should do it again," she responded quietly. "I'm glad we did it the first time. It helped her a whole bunch and gave her many months of good life. But to do it again wouldn't be for Tillie. It would be for me. It's not fair of me to ask that of her."

Later that week, I made my way to Lisa's house. She, Tillie, and Grizzly were behind the house, in the pasture down by the river. Destiny trotted around the fence line, no doubt expecting us to chase her down. When Grizzly saw me, he immediately squatted and peed in the grass. Tillie's head remained down, though her sad eyes tracked me across the pasture. She clearly felt awful, the whites of her eyes beginning to radiate the subtle yellow hue of jaundice, evidence that the cancer was now affecting the liver. Lisa's decision to put Tillie to sleep, though excruciating, had clearly been the right one.

It is an incredibly intimate thing to encroach upon the dynamics of an unraveling partnership, fleeting for the person, lifelong for the pet. But as a veterinarian, I have been invited into such a position innumerable times. It is a responsibility that never ceases to plunge me deeply into the substance of the bond between human hearts and the hearts of trusting and faithful animals. At no other time is the current of that bond more tangible to me, its waves washing over the aching people, crashing onto the unyielding rocks of the pet's illness and suffering, high tides of emotion eddying around the owners and the pet, their undercurrents pulling at me, too. The vulnerability of the people, the helplessness and dependence of the patient, the mortal significance of the owner's deliberations, the emotional consequences of a loathsome decision, the weight on my shoulders of my professional input all combine to make this event one of the most intensely difficult of professional interactions. But to do this for Lisa and Tillie produced an added layer of emotional expense.

Still, though all of these factors were present that afternoon in the field by the river, there remained in my mind an odd serenity that what I would do next would be a smoothly dove-tailed continuation of the care I had provided for Tillie and for Lisa. Together, we had faced the worst of medical diagnoses, the contemptible ogre, Cancer. Through the art and science of modern medicine, we had chased him away, his tail tucked like a coward, running from our poisons and persistence like some dangerous quarry that, when finally trapped, turned on us with vicious teeth and inflicted the mortal wound.

Our battle had been valiant, our purpose worthy. But in the end, the foe had been too vigorous. Fighting on would serve only to accentuate our own impotence and the overpowering might of the disease. The adversary could not be beaten. But the triumph of his conquest could be appropriated by stealing from him the right to decide the time and circumstances of his final victory. It was for us to choose how and when to ease the agony, to release the anxiety. We could administer the demise as we had administered the remedy. And this was a victory of sorts, a feeble finger in the eye of the evil monster. If the war must be lost, we could at least surrender on our own terms.

It was right that I was here in this field with Lisa and Tillie, Grizzly circling us with questioning and confused eyes. As Tillie slipped over the threshold of eternity, dignified and noble to the end, Lisa leaned her head against my shoulder. Grizzly sniffed the still form of his mother once, then turned to Lisa and licked the tears from her cheeks. My eyes filled with tears. I could feel my heart beating, could sense the blood surging through my veins with each contraction, an intricately choreographed dance by a million, a billion individual cardiac muscle cells even as Tillie's equally intricate heart stilled. Around this island of grief I could hear the bubbling of the river, the twittering of the warblers in the oak branches, the quiet rhythms of love drummed by a gentle hand on stilled ribs. I hoped those were the last things Tillie's ears heard, too.

Lisa chose to memorialize Tillie by engraving her name on the smoothness of a granite slab. That polished stone, its face level with the cold ground, was sunk into the grass in the shadow of a purple elm tree in Lisa's yard. It represented for Lisa the permanence of the impact Tillie had etched on her heart.

A Tick in Time

Mrs. Laughlin was . . . well, let's say unique. My first introduction to her was when I saw her dog for a bloody nose. Blimpie was a nondescript mongrel of the Labrador persuasion, with a short dark brown coat and ears that drooped. In fact, just about everything on Blimpie drooped, as he was extraordinarily appropriately named. So fat was Blimpie that it took two people heaving and grunting, to lift him onto the examination table. Weighing in at about seventy-five pounds, he was easily twice the dog he should have been. The impact of such an enormous mound of adipose tissue was compounded by the dripping of blood from his nostril, which had left blood on the floor, the walls, and the sides of the examination table by the time I entered the room.

And yet, despite the blood-soaked, crime scene–like room, it was Mrs. Laughlin who jumped out at me even more. Her figure, no less globoid than Blimpie's, strained and stretched the shiny fabric of her horizontally striped polyester blouse and slacks. She was in her late fifties, with hair dyed coal black. She sported oversized dark horn-rimmed glasses and entirely too much eye shadow. Her face, despite being heavily caked with foundation makeup, was hard and lined with stern creases. She talked incessantly and inanely.

What startled me most, however, were the violent twitches that ravaged her face every three to four seconds, the only things that seemed able to interrupt her nonstop chatter. They so jarred me that I found myself ignoring the obesity of my patient, the yards of polyester, and the dripping blood to focus on those facial contortions. Fortunately, Mrs. Laughlin didn't seem to notice. She was too occupied with concern for Blimpie to recognize my slack-jawed fascination.

Mrs. Laughlin was a frequent visitor to our hospital. She owned a number of dogs, which were the center of her rather small world and for whom she cared a great deal. Unfortunately, she lavished on them the same attention to healthy diet, exercise, and cleanliness that she afforded herself, and this necessitated frequent veterinary intervention.

I often wondered how her husband felt about the investment she made in her pets. I assumed from her wedding ring that she had a husband, though it was not until several months after my first exposure to Mrs. Laughlin that I actually met him. When I finally did, I understood for the first time that in this world there is someone for everyone.

The Laughlins made quite a pair. Mr. Laughlin was as thin as his wife was not. At six feet three and weighing only about 140 pounds or so, his clothes hung loosely from his sharp shoulders. His skin and hair seemed to do the same. While she jabbered incessantly, he rarely spoke. After years of heavy smoking, his voice, when he did speak, was throaty and choked, croaking out gravelly words in short bursts.

But Mr. Laughlin shared with his wife a common love for their dogs. He suffered her indulgences with amazing patience and unapologetic complicity. Once, after I had successfully treated Blimpie for an episode of disk disease and a painful back, he gripped my hand firmly and locked eyes with me in a steady, tear-laden gaze of gratitude before turning and leaving without a word. None was necessary.

One day, after I had become familiar with

the Laughlins, Mrs. Laughlin presented her dog Susie for evaluation of a cough. On examination, I found harsh, moist lung sounds, an irregular heart rhythm with a loud murmur, and a moist, choking cough. X-rays showed dramatic heart enlargement and fluid accumulation in the lungs. Susie was in congestive heart failure. I sat down with Mrs. Laughlin in the examination room. I knew that times were tough for the Laughlins financially, and she needed to hear the straight scoop.

"Mrs. Laughlin, things don't look good for Susie. Her heart is very large, and there is fluid leaking into her lungs as a result of poor heart function." I could tell by the increase in the frequency and severity of the facial twitching that the news was hitting home. Her face and neck were racked with nearly tetanic spasms.

"You know I take care of my dogs way too well, don't you, Dr. Coston?" Her verbal response belied her emotions. "I probably take better care of them than I do of myself or my husband."

I didn't find this difficult to believe. I could tell that Mrs. Laughlin needed a little time to process the news before coming back to the discussion at hand. Part of being a good veterinarian is sensing not only the medical needs of the patient but also the emotional needs of its owner.

"I know you love them very much," I said.

"That's right! You know I have five dogs."

"Yes, I've met them all."

"And not many people would let all five dogs sleep with them, would they?"

"You mean that all five dogs sleep with you?" I feigned surprise, thinking instead that few other living things would be interested. Trying to lighten the moment, I added without thinking, "I hope there's still room for your husband."

I knew instantly that this had been a mistake. One should not inadvertently open doors that one does not wish to walk through. And some people have no aversion whatsoever to barging through doors that should have remained closed and entering rooms where visitors should not be invited. If I had doubts about whether or not Mrs. Laughlin was one of these people, they were quickly erased as she pushed past me through the door I had opened.

"Heavens no! My husband and I haven't slept in the same room for years."

"Oh." I kept my voice deliberately disinterested, trying desperately to close the door behind her. "So . . ."

"No. He makes all those disgusting noises

when he breathes. They're so loud, I just can't sleep," she continued.

"Oh really?" I said flatly. "Now, back to Susie."

"No, we have separate rooms now. It really works out best that way. Good riddance, as far as I'm concerned." She pressed on, despite the fact that I was now putting Susie's X-rays up on the view box and pointing with my pen to the enormous heart framed by lungs that, because of the accumulated fluid, were altogether too white. "You know, just a few months ago my husband came to me and said he wanted to try it just one more time."

This was precisely the discussion I was trying to avoid. "Here are the X-rays I took of Susie this morning." I turned my back to her and tapped my pen tip on the films, as if to demonstrate a vitally important point.

Ignoring me completely, Mrs. Laughlin continued. "Even though I didn't think it was such a good idea, I finally gave in. But do you know what happened?"

I took a deep breath, turned back to her, and flopped into my seat with a sigh of resignation. I had only myself to blame for this; I was the one who had started it. But honestly, I had not expected her to plunge headlong into the room as she had done.

And, heaven knows, I had not expected her to turn the lights on.

"No, what happened?"

"Well, when he came into the room, Blimpie was lying on the bed. He bristled all up and started to growl at Jim. The closer Jim came, the more Blimpie growled. Why, he wouldn't even let Jim in the bed. Finally, Jim just gave up and left. Said something about it not being worth all that. And he hasn't tried again since then."

Choking back a laugh and quashing any temptation to ask further questions, I dived at the chance to gain control of the discussion again. Clearly, Mrs. Laughlin's own discomfort about this topic was not enough to veer her away from it, and the blushing awkwardness I was experiencing obviously hadn't occurred to her. I figured that perhaps she could be gently led away from it. This digression was, after all, only an excuse to avoid an even more uncomfortable and painful topic. I hoped a bit of gentle leading would work.

"Your husband hasn't been well lately, I've heard. Is that true?"

"Gracious yes. Jim's developed throat cancer and has had to have a tracheostomy tube placed. So he can't go out much anymore. Dr. Coston, you just wouldn't believe how much his medications cost us now. We're not wealthy people, you know. We're on Social Security and that's about all. It just about puts us under each time he has to get a prescription renewed. Sometimes we have to choose between drugs and food."

"That gets us back to Susie, Mrs. Laughlin. Her heart is not doing well at all." I waited to see if she was following my lead. She remained quiet, her eyes cast dejectedly to the floor, where Susie struggled for each breath.

"I just knew something was seriously wrong with her this time. She's almost thirteen years old this year. But I want you to do everything possible for her, Dr. Coston. She's all I've got." Mrs. Laughlin's voice cracked.

"I know she means a lot to you, Mrs. Laughlin. But she's not all you have. You have four other, younger dogs that are in pretty good shape. And you have a husband at home who needs you very much." I tried to provide some perspective for her. "Susie's condition is very serious. It is possible to use medications to try to help her heart function as efficiently as possible for as long as possible, but . . ."

"Good. I knew I could count on you to

make her better, Dr. Coston. That's just what I want you to do."

"Let me finish, Mrs. Laughlin. Medications may help, but it's also possible that we won't be able to improve her condition. And even if she does improve, it may be for only a short time. In the best of scenarios, maybe only a few weeks or months." I purposely painted a bleak picture for her, knowing that she would hear only the most rosy of predictions. For a moment, Mrs. Laughlin was uncharacteristically quiet, and I thought she was beginning to grasp the gravity of the situation.

"Now, I know how much she means to you," I continued, "but I also know that you've got to think about this in relation to all the other things you are facing right now, too. Maybe it wouldn't be in your best interest to pursue Susie's treatment aggressively right now. We could give her some medications to make her as comfortable as possible and . . ."

"I know what you're saying is right, Dr. Coston. But it's awful hard to think about it like that. I want to do everything I possibly can." I could sense the agony of the decision for her.

"I just don't want you to be in the position where your budget is stretched too tight for you."

"Don't you worry about that a bit, Dr. Coston. Money is no object. We're in pretty good shape financially, all things considered."

"Now, Mrs. Laughlin, you just told me that things were really tight with all of Jim's health-care costs. I know they can be exorbitant. And you shouldn't be forced to decide between buying medication for your husband or buying medication for Susie. Given those alternatives, your decision is a lot easier, don't you think?"

Mrs. Laughlin was quiet for a moment before shrugging noncommittally. "No, not really. Jim . . . he's almost gone anyway."

Clearly, Mrs. Laughlin was not able to process things objectively at this time. Someone would have to make a decision, and that someone had to be me.

"Okay. I'll tell you what I'm going to do. I'm going to prescribe some medications to try to pull some of the fluid from Susie's lungs. That should make her feel much better. I'll want to recheck her progress in a week. Can you do that?"

About a month later, Mrs. Laughlin brought in Blimpie for his annual vaccinations. She was strangely subdued. Her usually incessant blather was absent, though the violence of her facial contortions was not, and her face twisted into painful-looking spasms every few seconds. After Blimpie had received his shots and I had once again undertaken the fruitless task of instructing her on the benefits he would receive from calorie restriction, Mrs. Laughlin fixed me with an unusually vulnerable expression.

"Thank you, Dr. Coston, for your help with Susie. We did the right thing. You know, I lost Susie and my husband within a week of each other."

Her grief was clear and deep, and my heart went out to her. My mind replayed the profound sadness I had experienced many times at the passing of a beloved pet. I thought of my first dog, Thumper, and of Ollie and Rush. Such losses cut deep at the core of every animal lover. But the death of a spouse is a loss of a magnitude that I can neither conceive of nor bear to imagine. Mrs. Laughlin had faced both in the span of only one week. Nothing I could say to her, no matter how thoughtful or heartfelt, could offset the gravity of such pain.

A question played at the edges of my mind as I watched a tear make its way down the twitching face of Mrs. Laughlin that day. It was a question that I did not have the nerve to ask, one that would have been completely inappropriate to pose. Which loss had been the hardest for her?

As I stood at the desk and watched Mrs. Laughlin and Blimpie wobble up the sidewalk, one of the receptionists made an offhanded observation that summed up our impressions of her. "You just never know what makes some people tick, do you?"

SIALADENITIS

Mr. Johnston's name was on the appointment book for a problem with his cat, Thurgood. This was good and bad. From my previous interactions with him, I knew that an appointment with Mr. Johnston would always be entertaining, so distorted would be the dialogue. But over the years, his attitude had gone from mildly disdainful to blatantly disrespectful. This made for incredibly frustrating engagements. I was not looking forward to my appointment with Mr. Johnston, so later that morning, as I picked up Thurgood's record and made my way into the examination room, I took a deep breath of apprehension.

"Good morning, Mr. Johnston," I said, more cheerfully than I felt. I would try to overwhelm him with kindness, "How are you this fine morning?"

The uninterested, somewhat bored expression on his face remained unchanged by my greeting. "I'm not here for pleasantries, if you don't mind. I'm only here because something's not right with Thurgood."

"I'm sorry to hear that. What seems to be the problem?"

"He's showing a degree of unappetation. And he's usually a big eater."

"How long has that been going on?" I asked as I slipped a thermometer into my patient's rectum.

"Why, exactly, is it that you still insist on using those old-fashioned poobus thermometers?" His reddish face was cast in a pose of sheer ridicule, his unruly hair sliding down over his angry eyes.

"Because I haven't been able to get my patients to keep a thermometer under their tongues for two minutes yet," I responded, making a conscious effort not to respond in kind to his attitude.

"You do know they now have thermometers that you just insert into the ear, don't you?"

"Yes, I've tried those and found them not very accurate, I'm afraid. The old tried-and-true methods still work best for me." I heard the beeping of the digital thermometer and glanced at the readout, then let out an involuntary sigh.

"Is he pyrotechnic?"

"He is pyrexic, if that's what you mean," I responded, amused. "His temperature is 105.3 degrees. That's pretty high for a kitty. How long did you say Thurgood has been feeling bad?"

"I didn't say." Mr. Johnston clucked his tongue at me with a disgusted shake of his head. "But it's been about two weeks now."

"Okay. And what symptoms has he shown, besides not eating well?"

"Just lying around a lot more, less active, and less interested in things. The weird thing is, he's been hypersavlivating."

Mr. Johnston looked at me furtively, measuring my respect for his unparalleled mastery of medical terminology. I was in no mood to indulge silliness, especially from one I knew would just disparage me anyway.

"Hypersavlivating?"

"Yeah, you know. Drooling a lot!" he said, his voice dripping with contempt for my ignorance. "The saliva is really thick and vicious, and it just hangs from his mouth all the time."

"How can you tell his saliva is vicious?" I knew he meant viscous, but I resisted the temptation to draw attention to his mistake.

"Vicious means thick and sticky and slippery. You should look it up in your medical dictionary when you have a minute." He laughed derisively, pleased at his naked barb.

"Oh, you mean viscous. Vicious is something else entirely." I closed the noose with as much innocence as I could muster. "Let's take a look at his mouth."

I turned Thurgood to face me and lifted his chin with my hand. Sure enough, a ropy strand of thick, tenacious saliva hung from one corner of his mouth. I lifted his lip and found an area of reddened, enflamed, and swollen tissue around the opening of the salivary duct on his upper jaw, from which the saliva issued. Feeling carefully with my fingers, I could follow the course of the swollen duct as it made its way beneath the skin between the salivary gland and the opening in the mouth. Thurgood didn't like this probing, squirming in pain as I palpated the gland and the duct. For comparison, I repeated the exam on the opposite side. The duct there was not identifiable; the gland was painless.

"So what's the diagnosis?"

"Honestly, I'm not sure yet," I replied, puzzled. "I haven't seen this type of presentation before."

"I don't doubt that. I'm sure there are lots of things you don't know anything about."

"That's very true. But I didn't say I didn't

know what's going on. I said I had never seen this presentation before. I think this is a case of sialadenitis. And what you are seeing is ptyalism." It was time to fight fire with fire. If Mr. Johnston doubted my ability to throw around big words, it was time to lay his fears to rest. And it appeared that my efforts had their effect.

"Si . . . sinitis?" My salvo had found its mark.

"Sialadenitis. It means inflammation of the salivary glands. And I think that's what Thurgood has."

I remembered from my first meeting with Mr. Johnston and Dahmun that he considered himself a linguist and had invented his own language. Perhaps he would have been impressed to know that I had just invented this diagnosis, as well. The fact that I could support the term medically was beside the point. It was a descriptive that certainly fit. This was indeed inflammation of the salivary gland. But I had never before seen the term or the diagnosis printed in the veterinary literature. I was not familiar with a specific syndrome characterized by fever, glandular pain, and excessive salivation. I certainly did not know a cause or a treatment for this problem. Still, the terminology had hit its target and left this man speechless.

"Tie . . . a what?"

"Ptyalism. That's a medical term that means excessive salivation. That's the main symptom of Thurgood's sialadenitis." The word just seemed to flow off the tongue now, as if it was a diagnosis that I had dealt with every day for years, rather than one I had just invented.

"What causes it?"

"In Thurgood's case, I'm not sure. It isn't seen very often. With his fever, I suspect it's bacterial. I think we need to do a bacterial culture to see if that's the case."

I thoroughly swabbed the opening of the salivary duct with gauze until the hanging saliva strands were gone. Then I massaged the painful gland until more saliva began to flow. With a sterile swab, I dabbed at the duct's opening, coating the cotton swab with a layer of the slimy material, which I placed into bacterial medium. This I would send to the lab. Hopefully, it would identify whether there was a bacterial infection present and what antibiotic might be effective in eradicating it.

"So that's it?" Mr. Johnston snorted. "You're done?"

"Well, it will take about three or four days to get the results of the culture and sensitivity back. It won't be till then that we'll know exactly what's causing the problem and how to treat it."

"And Thurgood has to suffer until then?"

"I hope not. I will start some antibiotics and some medication for inflammation now. And I hope that will help him. But we may have to change the antibiotics once the culture results come back. I'll call you when they're here."

"Well, you should know that I'm not particularly pleased with your lack of expertise in this case."

And with that, Mr. Johnston took Thurgood home. I sent along a course of antibiotics for him to give Thurgood and a short course of anti-inflammatory drugs to relieve the discomfort. Four days later, I got the results of the culture and sensitivities back. A very aggressive bacterium was identified, one that was resistant to many types of antibiotics. Fortunately, the particular one that I had sent home with Mr. Johnston was effective.

At the recheck appointment two weeks later, I learned that Thurgood had recovered completely. No longer was he experiencing pain, and the swelling of the salivary gland and duct were resolved. His appetite had returned and his temperature was normal.

He was, in all respects, a completely normal cat again. Yet there was a palpable undercurrent of unhappiness as I discussed the case with Mr. Johnston. It was as if this near-miraculous response was a keen disappointment to him; as if he would have preferred his cat to still be suffering rather than have my diagnosis and treatment be right.

To this day, I have never had another case quite like Thurgood's. I cannot recall a patient with the same constellation of symptoms and physical findings. I have not since diagnosed bacterial sialadenitis, nor seen it in the journals. I still cannot explain exactly how or why Thurgood developed such an unusual problem. But I can look back on a successful outcome to a puzzling case. And there is much satisfaction in that.

For months, though, I seethed inside whenever I recalled the insolence and anger that Mr. Johnston had shown me during the management of Thurgood's illness. I could have understood the attitude had the patient not recovered completely, or had the medication caused some deleterious side effects. It might be forgiven if the bill had been excessively high or if I had been as hostile and argumentative to him as he had been to me. But none of that had been true.

It is a bit embarrassing how much the

frustration nagged at my mind. I vowed that if ever I was presented with one of Mr. Johnston's animals again, I would be assertive in addressing his demeaning and disrespectful attitudes, and this resolve brought a sense of closure to my troubled mind. Mr. Johnston's attitude faded from my attention.

My First Veterinary Technician

As the caseload in my nascent practice increased, I needed more help. True, I had a number of staff members by that time, receptionists and kennel attendants. I was no longer walking the dogs during the weekends or mopping the floors each morning. But I did find myself spending more and more time doing things that I could just as easily have delegated to others.

I was the only one, for instance, who could legally give injections, take X-rays, place intravenous catheters, induce anesthesia, or draw blood for laboratory testing. In Virginia, these tasks, many of which are similar to the tasks a nurse does in a human hospital, require education, training, and licensure. Since these were routine procedures in my office, it was necessary for me to devote a significant amount of my time to accomplishing them — time that I needed to commit instead to other patients. I needed a veterinary technician.

At this point in time, I cannot conceive of practicing without the assistance of veterinary technicians. Currently in our hospital, we employ five technicians. They are the ones who really allow my training and skills to blossom. I can see a patient, evaluate its condition, formulate a diagnostic plan of blood tests and X-rays, and prescribe a course of intravenous fluids and a smorgasbord of medications to treat the diagnosed condition. I then turn the patient over to my crack team of technicians and assistants and move on to my next patient. Their work makes my efforts a thousand times more efficient and increases exponentially the care provided to each patient.

When I was first starting out, though, I could not afford to hire a technician. Those tasks fell to me. This worked out okay for a while, when the caseload allowed me enough time to be a technician, as well. But my ability to treat my burgeoning number of patients efficiently was hampered by that lack as the practice grew.

This realization actually hit me full force one incredibly busy day as I was developing an X-ray in the darkroom. In those days, the job required a person to go into a closet-size room in absolute darkness and remove the X-ray film from the cassette, attach it to a metal frame, and dip it sequentially into the three tanks, which contained, respectively, the fixing, rinsing, and developing chemicals. It is much like a photographic darkroom process and requires that these things be done entirely by braille in almost palpable blackness. Because I could not open the door during the two or three minutes the X-ray was in the fixative and developer, the darkroom was often a haven for me during an incredibly busy and stressful day. Regardless of what was going on outside the darkroom door, I knew I had at least three minutes of uninterrupted calm. In the relaxation of complete darkness, I could, for a moment, completely empty my mind. I loved to develop X-rays.

It was at the beginning of this three-minute interlude that day when the receptionist banged on the door and informed me that a very serious emergency had just arrived unexpectedly and my presence was required in an exam room. No minutes ever went slower than those three minutes in the darkroom that day. Before I emerged to treat my patient, I had come to the unmistakable conclusion that I needed to hire a technician.

Unfortunately, knowing that you need to

hire one and actually doing so are two completely different animals. At that time in the state of Virginia, we were experiencing a significant shortage of veterinary technicians. The two schools in the state with vet-tech programs were graduating only about sixty or so graduates each year to fill the hundreds of slots in veterinary practices across the state. Most of the graduates were snatched up immediately by practices in larger cities and major metropolitan areas, where salaries were high. My chances of competing with those practices and attracting a technician to tiny little Woodstock were remote. Hourly wages for technicians in northern Virginia and the D.C. area were even higher than what I was able to pay myself at the time.

I placed a call to Dr. Potter, a friend and colleague of mine who headed a veterinary-technician program, one of two such programs in the state. He was not very encouraging, either. His graduates, he said, were in high demand and accepted positions often about a year in advance of their graduation dates. He had no current students who were not already committed to employment after graduation. He suggested that the best course of action would be for me to identify a worthy candidate among my staff to send to school, in the hopes that this person would choose to return to my practice after graduating.

"But that would mean more than a two-year delay in hiring a technician," I protested.

"You're right, Bruce, but I think that's your best hope," he replied. "And you'd better hurry. Applications for the next class are due next week. If you've got someone to send, you'd better get right on it."

Lisa came to mind even before I had put the receiver down. She had proved to be committed and responsible in her duties, duties that had grown as she had demonstrated her willingness to learn. But she also had some incredibly difficult challenges to consider. She had two children, one in elementary school and one in high school, who demanded a lot of time and attention. She also had very real financial constraints, which might make full-time schooling impossible. Finally, her background as a teenage mother who had not completed high school had left her with real self-esteem issues, which had hampered her ability to reach her potential. Still, I had confidence that all of these barriers could be surmounted if only she'd be willing to try. I called her into my office.

She came in with a look of concern on her face. Why was the boss bringing her into the office and closing the door? I motioned for her to take a seat, then fixed her with as enthusiastic a look as I could muster.

"Lisa, I think you have done a tremendous job since you joined our staff." She said nothing, her face a pillar of questions. "Are you enjoying your job?"

"Yes." Her response was tentative and guarded.

"Good. I've noticed that you are always willing to learn a new task and that you especially enjoy working directly with the medical aspects of the work."

"Uh-huh." She shifted uncomfortably in her seat.

"Do you see yourself continuing to be happy in your job?" I asked.

"I like my job a lot, if that's what you mean. I wouldn't want to lose it." Her face registered near panic.

"No, no, no," I said. "I don't want that, either. But I do see a larger role in the practice for you. Would you like that?"

"You mean a promotion?" She leaned forward in her chair.

"Well, yes. Absolutely a promotion," I replied. "Here's the thing. What would really help me a great deal would be to have a licensed veterinary technician whom I could lean on to do a lot of the technical things for the patients. A licensed technician could take X-rays, place catheters, give IV injections, induce and monitor anesthesia, do blood work, and manage patient care. Having someone who could do that would free up a lot of my time."

"Yeah, but I'm not licensed."

"Not now, but you could be."

"But doesn't that take a couple of years in college?"

"It is a two-year degree at a community college."

"But, Doc, I didn't even graduate from high school. I'm not a good student."

"You didn't graduate from high school because Melanie came along, not because you weren't a good student. And no, you didn't graduate, but you did get your GED, right?"

"Yeah, I did. But that was only because my mom pressed me on it." Anxiety edged Lisa's face, but it was an anxiety highlighted by a dawning of hope and eagerness. I pressed on.

"Lisa, it doesn't matter why you did it. The fact is, you did it. That means that you are qualified to apply to the veterinary-technician program. I've seen you work with the animals, and I've seen them respond to you. I think you could do it."

"They would never give my application a second look. I'd never get in."

"There certainly is that chance. But you never know till you try," I replied. "Besides, I happen to know the doctor in charge of the program quite well. I'll put in a good word for you. My guess is, they'll jump at you. You have experience at two veterinary hospitals. You have a level of maturity that most of their students don't have. And you have the full support of a veterinary hospital staff for your clinical work and the promise of a job coming out of school."

Lisa was quiet for a while. I watched her eyes wander around the room as she vacantly processed the million reasons why such a dream could never happen to her. On her face was such a mixture of excitement and fear that I wasn't sure whether she would jump up and hug me or run crying from the room. I let her mind grapple with the idea for a minute or two before proceeding.

"Lisa, you have so much more potential than being a kennel attendant forever. You're doing a great job at it and we're glad to have you here. But I see so much more you could do. I know it would be tough.

You'd have to travel the forty-five minutes to and from school each day. You would have to juggle your time to be a mom and a student. You'd have to figure out the finances of your schooling. You'd have to study your brains out. But I don't think any of those obstacles are insurmountable. I think you could do it. We can help you do it. And I could really use your skills in that role. I'd like you to pursue it. I want you to give it serious consideration."

"I don't know, Doc," she answered without conviction. "It sounds cool, but I'm just not sure. I will think about it, though. I'll get back to you in two or three weeks."

"You don't have two or three weeks. I've spoken with Dr. Potter at the school. The applications for this fall's class are due in one week. Think about it overnight and we'll talk tomorrow." I handed her a sheaf of papers with information about the career and the program. She left my office, shaking her head in bewilderment, unable to process the possibility that she might be in college that fall.

But the next morning, she was the picture of resolve. She had considered my suggestion seriously and had discussed it with Steve, her kids, and her mother. All of them had been enthusiastic about the possibility, offering to help out with the housework, the yard work, and the studying. Her mother had graciously offered to help with the tuition as much as possible. One by one, the barriers she thought were so towering had evaporated. She came in to my office first thing and settled confidently into the chair, her chin up and determination inhabiting her features.

"I've decided to give it a shot," she said. "But I'm going to need your help on a few things."

"Anything I can do."

"I might need your help getting my application together."

"I already had Dr. Potter fax me the forms. You can fill them out today and we'll go over them together."

"I need a letter of recommendation from you."

"I'll write you a doozy of a recommendation. They won't dare pass you up after they read my letter." Lisa laughed.

"Okay. Also, I think I'm going to need to continue to work part-time during school."

"I was hoping you would."

"And I might need some coaching and tutoring. I haven't been in school in a long time."

"I'll be glad to help with any of that you

might need. But I bet you won't need as much as you think."

"Well, I'm going to go for it, but I'm just going on the record now to say that I think my chances are slim."

"On the contrary, my friend. I think your chances are great! Only your confidence is slim."

It took Lisa most of the week to complete the application process. With little help from me, she wrote a compelling essay on why she would be a good technician, pulling from her experience working with sick pets. She outlined the type and extent of her exposure to the profession during the time she had spent as an employee, detailing the cases she had seen, the surgeries she had observed, and the work she had done. Her time with us far exceeded the fifteen or twenty hours of observation required of applicants, placing her in the upper echelon of candidates. I contributed a stellar endorsement of her professionalism and skills in my letter of recommendation. I was confident that she would be given strong consideration.

The two months between when the applications were due and when the candidates were accepted was inordinately long for Lisa. I maintained that her acceptance was a foregone conclusion. But Lisa spent the time in anxious, lip-biting anguish. I did note that just the process of outlining her accomplishments for the admissions committee endowed Lisa with a new flush of confidence and optimism. There was a fresh level of interest in each case, a renewed commitment to the needs and comfort of each patient, and an invigorated approach to interacting with the clients and her coworkers. Goals do that for a person.

I must admit here to a bit of foreknowledge. Dr. Potter contacted me about some other business, and during our conversation he let slip the fact that the admissions committee had selected Lisa to be in the upcoming class of veterinary technicians. I knew the outcome two weeks before Lisa did. But I kept quiet. I did not want to spoil for her the joy of opening that letter of acceptance. Nor did I want her to think that I had interceded on her behalf and convinced the committee, against their better judgment, to give her a chance. I had not. She had been accepted on her own merits, without any input from me. It was her triumph and I did not want to diminish it in any way. But that was a difficult secret to keep as I watched Lisa's nails get bitten shorter and shorter.

When the letter did arrive, Lisa's sense of success and achievement was beyond my expectation. To see the jubilation of accomplishment on her face as she laid the envelope on my desk was a thing of beauty. With glistening eyes, she listed the things she needed to do before the fall semester started. It would be work, but I could tell that a fire of pride and accomplishment had been kindled in her heart. She turned to me before she left the office.

"Doc, I would never have thought this was possible. I can't thank you enough for encouraging me to give this a try. I won't let you down."

"I have no doubt of that, Lisa. You're going to do great."

And she did. She was not a straight A student, but her grades were respectable, and though she tended not to test well, she clearly knew the material. I saw her training reflected in her job performance. Her part-time work took on a much more serious and clinical approach, a change that benefited the patients and set a good tone for the rest of the staff. As she learned more about specific techniques, she brought that knowledge to bear on each animal she worked with. Her classes provided her the opportunity to understand the significance of the tests and techniques she had helped me with for years.

As her medical-knowledge base increased, so did her confidence and sense of self. She became more and more assertive in dealing with clinical situations and directing the efforts of the staff. Her interactions with the clients reflected this change, too. In no time, she grew well beyond my limited expectations.

Between her first year of school and her second, she was required to complete an internship in the clinical context of a veterinary hospital. She spent the summer with us, of course, honing her skills. I quickly began to rely on her growing arsenal of clinical tasks and knowledge. Tillie's disease had provided her a special reason to nourish an interest in treating cancer patients, and this skill was put to use that summer in treating a number of patients so afflicted.

Before I knew it, Lisa's schooling was coming to an end. She took and passed her national and state board exams, the culmination of her training and the gates through which every technician must pass to enter the profession. I received a graduation announcement in the mail one day. Graduation day for her was a cool Saturday afternoon in May. With an almost paternal sense of pride, I watched Lisa march down the aisle in her cap and gown. She had accomplished a nearly miraculous transformation since my first introduction to her — truly a caterpillar to butterfly metamorphosis. From that quiet, self-conscious, and timorous person had emerged this confident, skilled, and intense woman of achievement and resolve. Even her physical movements reflected this change, her strides confident and purposeful as she walked to the front, the tassel swinging from her mortarboard.

You don't often have the chance to witness the rebirth of a person; to stand in awe and respect as someone sheds the chrysalis constructed from the baggage of circumstance, of poor decisions, of economic entrapment, of faded dreams or psychological inertia. Such a personal reinvention requires of one a degree of courage and discipline that is wholly other than what life's routine becomes. It is not a fight-or-flight, heedless act of courage in the face of imminent danger, the instinctual aggression of a protective mother, brave as that might be. It insists instead upon a complete review of all possibilities, a stern accounting of oneself, a thoughtful consideration of every contingency, including failure, that such a change might bring. It involves the cognitive ejection of all hindrances to progress, be they behaviors, attitudes, relationships, or indulgences. This intimidating process is one that, in many, grinds personal development to a quaking and pitiful halt. The inevitable stretching and pulling and testing leaves one strengthened and ennobled. It is uncomfortable, to be sure, but the product is personal achievement and accomplishment that builds success upon success, etching into one's core an immutable sureness.

This is what I saw in Lisa's eyes that day as she shook Dr. Potter's hand and grasped with eagerness her diploma. And though I knew her achievements were her own, I still took a bit of pride in the moment, as well. After the ceremony, as her family gathered around her in celebration, I joined them on the lawn. She turned to me with her new-found confidence and fixed me with a steady look.

"Thank you, Doc," she said, grabbing my hands and holding my eye.

"Lisa, you did this on your own. You didn't need any help from me."

"You're right: I completed it. But you sparked the interest in it. You goaded me to try. I wouldn't have done it without you."

"Don't cut yourself short, Lisa. It took a lot of resolve to do it," I responded. "Besides, it was purely selfish of me."

"What do you mean by that?"

"I fully expect to have a licensed veterinary technician till death do us part!" I joked, blissfully unaware of the prescient irony.

Lisa laughed and gave me a huge hug. "Deal!"

Unwelcome Appointment

It wasn't the quiet chuckle that died abruptly as I walked through the door that got my attention. I just assumed I'd come in too late to hear the latest inside joke between the receptionists. It wasn't the way the conversation spontaneously went from boisterous to muted upon my entrance. I'd given careful instructions to the staff about how hushed conversations at the front desk are not professional. It wasn't even the mirthful glances that were my first clue. It was the subtle twinkle of mischief that hid in Rachel's eyes that day and that played furtively at the corners of her mouth. Those hints should have tipped me off. I should have known that Rachel was up to something.

But honestly, as the only man in an office full of women, there are a lot of interpersonal subtleties that elude me. I am usually the last to recognize that a tempest has blown up in the teapot of the office, even when the eye of the storm tracks directly over me. Whatever the cause of my oblivion, I completely missed the cues that day, distracted by the messages she handed me from clients who had called while I had been at lunch. It is only in retrospect that I now realize I should have known.

Besides, Rachel is the last person I would have suspected. She is an unassuming, quiet woman who, having worked in the office as a receptionist for many years, I know quite well. She is a remarkably proficient receptionist, one whom the clients love and who diligently goes about her duties. She was in her late twenties at the time and married, with a daughter and a fascinating personal history full of unexpected ironies. Her personality is very settled, with few emotional swings and a wit that is keen but subdued. She is one of those people you think you know well but whose waters run deep and unseen, with surprising turns and eddies, which become evident most easily when viewed from farther downstream than while passing over them.

"Mrs. White wants you to call her right away. Frosty has had diarrhea for a few days now and she is worried," she said as she handed me a phone message and Frosty's record.

"Did she not want to come in?" I knew Frosty was a tiny Maltese and it wouldn't take long before he was seriously dehydrated from persistent diarrhea.

"She will, but she wants to talk with you first."

"Okay, I'll call her. Anything else?"

"Yeah, guess who I just made an appointment for?" Rachel's smile revealed altogether too much enjoyment. I felt my guard go up, but I wasn't sure why.

"Who? Is it a client I'll be glad to see?"

"Mr. Johnston!" Now Rachel was laughing.

"No way! Not Mr. Johnston," I responded.

There are clients whose appearance on the schedule raises the spirits of everyone in the office. They are people who sweep joyfulness along in their wake, washing it over all those they encounter. These people usually have pets with the same delightful attitudes, and their effect on the staff is an amazing thing, infectious and uplifting. Then there are people like Mr. Johnston, whose presence blankets the environment with a critical and dissatisfied air of heaviness, one that is toxic with disdain and polluted with scorn. This attitude, too, has a predictable effect on the staff and poisons my own outlook.

"When is his appointment?"

"Two weeks from this Thursday."

"That's just great," I said in a tone of voice that communicated just the opposite. "Oh well, at least I won't have to worry about him for a couple of weeks. I'll go call Mrs. White about Frosty now."

I turned my attention to the other tasks at hand. There were patients in the hospital, surgeries to do, calls to make, clients to see. These all took my attention and occupied my time. But it would not be true to say that I did not worry about my upcoming appointment with Mr. Johnston. The truth is, It was always there as a nagging presence in the back of my mind. I knew I would have to suffer Mr. Johnston's negativity and pessimism, his lack of confidence in me, his disrespect and rudeness. I would somehow have to buffer the staff from his bullying and demeaning manner. The thought hung on like a virus, or the persistent cough after a bout of bronchitis.

Rachel didn't help matters any, either. Every other day, it seemed, she reminded me of the appointment. Sometimes it was with a laugh, as if she enjoyed the stress this was causing me. Sometimes it was with apparently the same dread that I felt, and she'd bemoan the emotional terrorism that she knew awaited her as a "lowly" receptionist. Many people who are civil, even friendly, with the doctors turn a nasty side to the receptionists. But Mr. Johnston was an equal-opportunity beast. He would berate both me and the staff equally — and seem to enjoy it.

"We've taken a survey and decided that you should be the one to deal with Mr. Johnston when he comes in," she said one day, a week or so before his appointment.

"Oh, yeah?" I replied. "Why, is everyone afraid of him?"

"There is just no reason why we should be treated badly by him. We don't get paid enough for that kind of abuse."

Neither do I, I said to myself. In fact, there wasn't enough money to compensate for the blatant disregard for common courtesy that Mr. Johnston displayed.

As I did routine surgeries, my mind was occupied with thoughts of Mr. Johnston and how to best handle his appointment. While I had purposed to be assertive, such confrontations do not come easily for me. I am one who loathes conflict. Attracting bees with honey is a much more comfortable tack for me. But I had already tried to overwhelm him with cheerfulness and that had failed miserably. I figured perhaps it would be better simply to keep the interaction on a strictly professional basis to minimize his chances of turning the conversation to personal things. Yet I knew from past experience that he would as quickly attack my professional skills as my personal failings, so that strategy provided me little cover, either.

These thoughts jumbled around in my head till nothing made sense and I felt silly for investing so much energy in hypothetical exercises. Why did Mr. Johnston even matter to me anyway? He was just an unhappy person whose personal approach to life I could not alter. Why let this one person so dominate my thoughts? There were, after all, lots and lots of clients who were loyal to the office and completely satisfied with our services. The management gurus tell us that fewer than 20 percent of clients are responsible for 80 percent of the complaints and that we should not allow that unhappy 20 percent to determine our approach and outlook with everyone else. Good advice! But difficult for me to internalize with Mr. Johnston's appointment looming.

This internal conversation persisted, on

and off, for the entire two weeks I knew Mr. Johnston had an appointment scheduled. Finally, on the day before the dreaded appointment, Rachel struck again.

"Tomorrow's the day, you know."

I knew without hesitation what she was referring to. I had been counting down the days in my brain, like an appointment with the IRS auditor.

"Which animal is he bringing in?" I asked.

"I don't remember, but it's one of the cats. I pulled the record today for tomorrow's appointment and remembered that he's one of your favorite clients." She chuckled. Apparently, she was enjoying my discomfort.

"Hardly. I've thought of little else since you told me about the appointment two weeks ago. I've about got myself worked up to an ulcer. I'll just be glad when it's over."

Why it was that I simply didn't call him up and cancel the appointment is beyond me now. But the thought had not entered my mind. I had charted a theoretical course through this minefield. But even up to that fateful morning, I had not decided exactly how I was going to handle Mr. Johnston.

As I showered that morning, though, I rehearsed a carefully worded speech that I would deliver to him when I first entered the examination room. Lathering my hair and soaping down my body, I edited and rehearsed the speech till I could say it without hesitation or apology.

I'd start it out nonchalantly. "Hello, Mr. Johnston. I'd like to talk over something with you before we get started today to make sure this appointment is successful for both you and me. It's been my observation over the years that we at Seven Bends Veterinary Hospital have often not been able to meet your expectations. This has apparently been very frustrating for you, judging by the way you interact with my staff and me. You should know this is very frustrating for us, as well. We want to provide the best care we possibly can for your animals and develop a relationship with you built on mutual respect. You can be sure that we will commit our best efforts on behalf of your pets. We will do it with care and compassion, and we will be sure to communicate with you exactly what is needed and why along the way. This we are committed to."

In my mind's eye, I could see him beginning to get uncomfortable. At that point, it would go one of two ways. Either he would fold and crumple into compliance like most bullies or he would get belligerent. I was prepared for either response. I would hold my hand up in a gesture of calm and continue.

"Let me finish, Mr. Johnston. This is important for us to get clear. I will promise you to do all those things. But you must promise me a few things, as well. For your part, you must promise to interact with us in respectful ways. It is neither fair nor acceptable for you to demean our efforts, our knowledge, and certainly not our compassion. It is not acceptable for you to criticize me or my staff while you are in this office. If we are unable to meet your expectations, I will be glad to provide your pets' medical records to a veterinary hospital that can. But it is important to me that I have relationships with my clients that are based on trust and respect. And if I am unable to earn your trust and respect, it's probably better for both of us for you to find another vet. Is that a fair request?"

It was a long speech for me to memorize. But over the course of two weeks, I had considered all the options, and this one seemed to be the best. I had parsed every sentence. I would be assertive but not rude. I would set ground rules for our continuing professional relationship that would be positive for both him and me. This would give him a way to opt out gracefully if he wished. It was the best I could do, but it still made me nervous.

The drive to the hospital that morning was clouded with concern over the impending interaction. The Bradford pear trees lining the streets of Woodstock were in full bloom. In flower beds in front of homes and businesses, the crocuses and daffodils had pushed through their blankets of mulch and were unfolding their colors to the springtime morning sunshine. On the shoulders of the Massanuttens, the trees were leafed out with their early spring green, fresh and vibrant, not yet the duller, darker green of summer. Unfortunately, these harbingers of spring escaped me as I drove, so involved was my mind with the task before me.

So it was with this sense of purpose and plan, overshadowed by acrid foreboding, that I walked into the clinic that morning. Mr. Johnston's appointment was the first on the book and I was ready. That was a good thing, too, because just a few minutes after I arrived at the hospital, Rachel found me.

"Mr. Johnston's here with his cat. And he's already ticked off. Good luck with this one." And she handed me his record.

I took a couple of minutes to go over the

speech again in my mind, cementing the most important points in my brain before going into the room. Then I took a deep breath of resolve and pushed the door open.

Confusion was the first impression I had. Nothing was as I'd expected it. Where was Mr. Johnston? I had expected to meet a surly, angry man with unkempt hair, but there was no one in the room. Sitting on the examination table was a stuffed teddy bear with a bandage on his leg. Around his neck hung an index card with writing on it, tied in place with red yarn. My mind struggled to understand the scene. What was going on? I pulled the door partially closed and looked behind it, half-expecting to find Mr. Johnston lurking there as he had been lurking in my mind for the past two weeks. But he was not. Bending down so I could see the writing on the index card, I noticed in the periphery of my vision movement behind me in the hall. What was written on the card? It hung so the writing was not immediately visible to me. I turned the card and pulled it closer so I could make out the words.

"APRIL FOOLS'!"

For a moment, the words made no sense to me. But then hooting began behind me, and I turned to find that my entire staff had mustered in the hall and were now cheering and laughing at me good-naturedly. Slowly, reality began to dawn. It was indeed April 1. I had been had!

I looked around at the small group of people enjoying the prank in the hallway. At the front was Rachel, laughing uproariously. It hit me at that moment. She was the one! She had conceived it, planned it, orchestrated every detail, and implemented it to perfection. It had been Rachel who had brought it up to me every other day, who had planted ideas in my head, who had fueled my fears and stoked the fires of drama. Rachel, of all people! My estimation of her climbed a few notches for the sheer chutzpah required to pull this prank off.

I began to laugh with them — in appreciation for the beauty of a plan well laid, in celebration of the camaraderie that fostered fun like this, in gratitude that my staff trusted me to respond appropriately. I laughed for all these reasons, yes. But to be honest, there was also the unburdening mirth of great relief. I would not have to see Mr. Johnston after all!

THE CORONATION OF THE QUEEN

Practically every veterinary hospital has a hospital mascot. These are usually rescue cats that Good Samaritans drop off for veterinary care or are patients whose owners discard them at the office, never intending to pick them up again. Veterinarians and their staffs are invariably good-hearted people who would rather gnaw off their own limbs than put such a kitty to sleep.

My own office is no exception. We have a long history of successive monarchs, Cy being the first. You may remember Cy if you read *Ask the Animals.* Cy's story came full circle on the very day of her passing when a little gray kitty was presented to the office for euthanasia, a coincidence that happened to be very much in her favor. No one in the office that day had the heart to put another cat down, especially one who could benefit from a little love and attention. She became the next hospital mascot. That little gray

175

kitten, like Cy, had to have one eye removed due to severe upper respiratory disease and the subsequent rupture of the globe. Because her circumstances were so similar to Cyclops's, we named her Ditto. She was the second queen of the office.

Even though Ditto was missing an eye, her beautiful gray color, rich lustrous coat, and diminutive size made her an endearing figure in the hospital after Cy's passing. It was fun to watch her grow, displaying the wonderful antics that make kittens so irresistible. The hospital staff was quickly drawn in by her. As an adolescent, she submitted without complaint to all the care kittens require in their first year. She went through her series of vaccines, let us collect stool and blood samples, and treat her ears for mites, her skin for fleas, and her intestines for worms. She even sailed through her surgical sterilization without batting her eye.

As a kitten, she made a bold statement to the clients when they saw the little bundle of gray energy on the reception desk. They, too, thought she was beautiful and showered her with attention. The kids, especially, wanted to hold her and hug her and carry her around the lobby. But as time went on and Ditto grew older, we realized she had one huge disadvantage that might compromise her success as a hospital mascot: She was gray!

I have found that certain generalizations hold true in cats of a certain stripe. Siamese cats, for instance, tend to be excessively vocal, tuxedo cats are usually people-oriented, and Ragdolls are extremely docile. Call me a racist if you must, but I have found that gray cats tend to be — how can I put this delicately? — psychotic.

I do not say this lightly. I happen to have a much-loved gray cat who, I must admit, has definite behavioral tendencies for which psychoactive drugs may eventually be necessary. I do know there are exceptions to the rule, so please spare me the angry letters that are being composed in your mind as you read this. This tendency is so often seen, though, that in our office, it has come to be known as the "gray cat syndrome."

When a gray cat comes into the office and displays stereotypical fractious behavior at the slightest provocation, gray cat syndrome is diagnosed and leather gloves and thick towels are often necessary. You might argue that the insertion of a thermometer into a tightly closed sphincter might provoke any rational being, gray or otherwise. But lots of tuxedo kitties and Ragdolls tolerate this invasion of their personal space with dignity and do not lash out with claws, teeth, and venom or fill the air with vile volleys of volatile verbiage the way gray cats routinely do.

Gray cats suffer from a common paranoia, an inexplicable deficiency of self-esteem that eventually renders many of them virtually incapable of interacting in constructive ways with others. They seem convinced that everyone around them, human or otherwise, is bent on their immediate demise — probably in cruel and painful ways. Thus their response is one of extreme defensiveness, even in the face of unexpected kindness. This constant state of self-preservation leaves them anxious and fidgety, like an untreated ADD sufferer, flitting constantly from one life-threatening emergency to another. Sudden noises, unexpected movements in their peripheral vision, unwelcome advances from strangers — even friendly ones — or an interaction with another animal shoots their stress hormones to untenable levels and induces in them behaviors that are counterproductive. Some get fractious. Some become sullen and withdrawn. Some develop behavioral disorders, making matters even worse.

Ditto, as I may have mentioned, was a

gray cat and therefore subject to gray cat syndrome. As you might imagine, a veterinary hospital is exactly the environment where such cats are exposed to all the circumstances on the above list and more. With time, Ditto's gray cat syndrome became more pronounced. Her strategy to deal with the stress, following the "misery loves company" dictum, was to create stress in others by threatening any client who dared to approach her. This was confusing to the clients, many of whom had known her as a kitten when she actively sought their attention. As she got older, though, her warnings to too-friendly clients became progressively more assertive, changing from a simple angry swishing of the tail to a noncommittal hiss and finally to a full-throated cry of rage.

Adults at whom this venom was directed were quick to withdraw. But children are more persistent with their rapprochement. We became concerned that one day Ditto might actually hurt one of them. The fact that Ditto might be happier in an environment other than a veterinary hospital began to slowly dawn on me. I broached this concept with the staff one day during our monthly meeting, only to be greeted by the human equivalent of gray cat syndrome from the majority of them.

In an effort to keep Ditto in the environment to which she had become accustomed, I decided that declawing her was necessary to prevent injury to unsuspecting clients. I know mentioning this procedure will bring out the ire of many a cat lover. I have faced this principled stance from cat advocates on many occasions, staring down indignant crusaders who have accosted me for performing the procedure on my patients. I, of course, share their obvious concern about inflicting upon undeserving animals a painful procedure that is merely for the convenience of uncaring people. It is true that some patients who have undergone declawing procedures have suffered horribly as a result of poorly done surgeries. It is also incontrovertible that declawing is not a normal procedure and changes forever the anatomy of the cat.

But in my experience, I have found that there are situations in which declawing a cat can save a threatened relationship with a loving family. For some people who suffer from diseases like diabetes or cancer or AIDS, which diminish their ability to fight off infections, a cat scratch can be a very serious thing indeed. Others face the obstacle of living with people who are not cat-oriented who would insist upon banishing the cat to the outdoors or getting rid of it entirely if even the slightest damage were to be inflicted on expensive furniture. In my view, it would be far crueler to sentence a cat to a lifetime of isolation from the family it loves than to have it declawed by a caring professional who does the procedure well and provides the patient with adequate pain control. Certainly you would agree with me that this is a better outcome than for the cat to be abandoned at the local shelter, where adoption rates are low and euthanasia rates are not.

And no, it is not normal to remove the claws of a cat. But the same people who harangue on this point are the first to belittle you if you fail to have your cat spayed or neutered; and it is no more normal to remove a uterus or a pair of testicles than to remove claws. Both surgeries are painful procedures, and I have seen as many patients suffer terribly from a spay or neuter gone awry as from poorly done declawing.

So, in an effort to salvage Ditto as the hospital mascot, she was declawed, a procedure that resulted in no long-term effects on her, though it failed to achieve its purpose. In the end, Ditto sabotaged our every effort to rehabilitate her. The last straw came when her psychosis evoked the unforgivable offense of inappropriate urination. Technically, it was not the inappropriate urination that damned her, but the inappropriate location in which she habitually chose to relieve herself — my briefcase.

Ditto was simply not happy in the helter-skelter world of the hospital. Fortunately, I was able to find her a home where the pace was slower, and her stress was greatly relieved. Reverend Cheaver, a quiet and dignified client whom I knew to be a devoted pet lover, agreed to welcome Ditto into his home.

In the dozen years or so since she left our hospital, I have provided Ditto's medical care free of charge. She is now a respectable senior citizen of about fourteen years of age. She has been under my knife to remove a hyperactive thyroid gland and is fed a special diet for her failing kidneys. But she is a happy geriatric cat, free of the many psychological demons that plagued her as an inmate of Seven Bends Veterinary Hospital. Like a parole officer, I see Ditto fairly often. Each time, she still cringes and hides, screams and swears when she sees me. Perhaps it is because she, too, thinks of me as a parole officer. But Ditto remains to this day a gray cat, complete with all the psychological accoutrements that so often accompany those with her coloration; so I suspect her bad attitude is more likely a symptom of gray cat syndrome.

It was several months after Ditto joined the Cheaver family that another monarch came to the throne. This time it was the work of a Good Samaritan. One of the local workers at the regional Health Department brought in an adolescent cat he had picked up on the road after seeing it get hit by a car in a nearby county. He had first taken it to another veterinary hospital, where the cat had been diagnosed with head trauma and discharged with antibiotics and instructions to bring him back in two or three weeks to be castrated.

When the cat was still not walking five days later, the kind gentleman brought it to me for a second opinion. The cat was mostly white, with patches of brown tabby splashed haphazardly across its sides, back, and head. Its face was distorted by a badly broken canine tooth, which pointed forward like a hood ornament through parted and bloody lips. Damage to the bones around the lower jaw and lips had left the mouth skewed and painful. The cat was alert and followed my every move with bright and soulful eyes, but it could barely keep itself righted as it sat heavily on its chest, its front legs splayed awkwardly to each side. When I lifted the cat into a standing position, it was able to bear weight on its hind legs, but both front legs hung limply, refusing to cooperate with the cat's obvious intentions. Each time the cat tried to place weight on her legs, it crumpled pitifully onto its little nose, leaving a bloody spot on the table where the injured tooth and lips hit.

The cat's left leg buckled painfully between the elbow and shoulder, and the kitty flinched noticeably when I felt in that region with gentle fingers. Any manipulation of the dangling leg resulted in a grating of bone, which sent little shivers of pain through the cat's body. I knew in an instant that the leg was fractured. X-rays would be required to identify the severity of the break, but I was confident that surgery would most likely be necessary to stabilize the fracture enough for healing to take place. This was a major injury.

The cat's right leg sagged limply at the elbow, the toes knuckling over, so the top of the foot rubbed on the ground. It had no strength to hold weight or to resist my manipulations of the foot. The fact that progressively firmer squeezes of the toes failed to evoke even the slightest response from the cat indicated that the sensory and motor nerves of that leg had suffered severe trauma. I had seen this type of injury before. It is termed brachial plexus avulsion and means that the brachial plexus, essentially the major neurologic relay station for the nerves serving the front leg, has been damaged. It is an injury from which many cats do not recover. A percentage may, with the passage of a few weeks or months, regain a measure of neurologic function in the leg, but many are left with permanently non-functional limbs, which must later be amputated. This, too, is a life-changing trauma.

The rest of the examination was anticlimactic, though I was surprised to identify a series of soft egg-size water balloons in the cat's abdomen and a small amount of blood that had collected in the hair under its tail. Contrary to what the man had been told, this was not a male cat; in fact, it was soon to be the mother of four kittens. Because of her massive injuries, I knew the likelihood that she would carry the litter to term was low — especially with the presence of blood.

I'm not sure what had distracted the veterinarian who initially evaluated the cat that day. Heaven knows, I am not always at the top of my game. But his diagnosis for this patient could not have been further from the mark had it been made by a four-year-old with a Magic 8 Ball. And because of his missed diagnosis, this cat had suffered miserably for five days. I was steamed!

The reasonable thing would have been to put the hurting and confused kitty out of its misery. There was no hovering and worried owner to provide the cat's necessary aftercare. Neither was there anyone stepping forward to cover the costs of the extensive surgeries that would almost certainly be required. The Good Samaritan who had brought her to us made it clear that he was not in a position to take the cat himself and that he would understand completely if our recommendation was an irrevocable one. But, though these considerations were valid, when I looked into that little cat's trusting eyes, rationality gave way to empathy.

This cat had already been failed by my profession. It seemed somehow too cruel to have imposed on her five days of needless suffering only to give up on her now. She had not deserved to be left alone to care for herself. She had not deserved to become a teenage parent. She had not deserved to be struck by a car. She had not deserved to be misdiagnosed and left untreated. After we had failed her on so many counts, she did not now deserve to be discarded like so much unwanted feline rubbish.

Despite her debilitating injuries, the cat was exceptionally friendly and trusting, head-butting me and purring loudly as my mind surveyed the options. The broken left leg would have to be repaired with a major orthopedic surgery requiring weeks of recovery. The right leg, I was sure, would eventually have to be amputated. But that could wait for six or eight weeks while her broken bone mended. The dangling tooth would have to be extracted and some reconstructive work would need to be done to the lips and jaw. She would also need to be spayed.

I knew the care for this unwanted cat could easily top $2,500, an amount I knew I would not recover. But something about this cat had already staked a claim on me, and a quick glance at Susan and Lisa made it clear that they had also been affected. The hesitation and indecision on my face did not go unnoticed.

"You know," began Susan, "we don't have a hospital mascot anymore now that Ditto's gone. This cat would make a great blood donor."

"And the clients always warm up to a disabled cat," added Lisa, her eyes a plea.

"Somehow, I just can't make myself put this cat down," I said. "Let's get some blood for testing and see where this goes."

Where it went was a rerun of what had transpired with previous rescue kitties. When I pointed this out to Susan and Lisa, they agreed so completely that we immediately began to call her Rerun. It was a name that stuck. I took her to surgery the next day and repaired her broken bone with pins and wires, removed her tooth, repaired the damage to her jaw and face, and spayed her. It was a marathon of unreimbursed surgery. But the rewards were immediate and measured in currency of more value than legal tender. It is, in fact, an investment that is still paying dividends.

Rerun's personality blossomed as soon as the intractable pain from the broken bone was addressed. She was playful and endearing, despite being hampered by the useless leg, which she dragged along beside her. Because she could not limp on both front legs simultaneously, she began using the operated leg right away.

Lisa was right. The clients loved Rerun. She was an immediate hit! There's something irresistible about a pathetic invalid. She warmed to this new role like a starlet to the lights. Within just a week or so, it was clear that she would be a permanent fixture in the office.

She displayed none of Ditto's angst, loving the hectic, busy pace and the constant flow of the dogs and cats that moved like slow breaths in and out of the hospital. She would perch herself on the reception desk and survey each new patient with studied indifference. Some seemed to catch her attention more than others, though I could not discern what spurred her interest in specific animals. It was unrelated to size, gender, or species. She was just as likely to be drawn to a big, imposing dog as to a cat. If anything, she showed more interest in the dogs than in her own peers. When a new patient interested her, she would jump down off the desk and sidle up to it, tail high and leg dragging, to sniff its nose before walking away, apparently satisfied.

One day about three weeks after her surgery, I was surprised to notice that Rerun was subtly advancing her right foot forward and placing it on the ground with the pads down rather than simply dragging the tops of the toes behind her. At first, I thought my eyes were deceiving me, so subtle was the change. But over a period of a few days, it was clear that she was beginning to regain some neurologic function in the leg. Slowly, the improvement continued, till finally there was no hint left of the neurologic trauma she had sustained.

Rerun is still a beloved presence in our practice. This year she will pass her twelfth year with us. Her reign, which began with frantic energy and nonstop activity, has now settled into a calm and controlled routine. The clients know her well and look for her at each visit. Her tangle with the automobile as a young stray has left its mark. With time, the right foot has steadily and progressively deviated outward, so that she now walks with those toes pointed to the side, as if to signal a turn. The strain this places on her joints has left her with marked arthritis, for which she is treated with glucosamine, anti-inflammatory medication, and periodic acupuncture therapy.

She has earned her keep over the years by providing comic relief to waiting clients and overworked staff, by acting as an unpaid welcoming committee, and by occasionally donating blood to anemic patients, a role she would rather avoid. But her life has been full. As a senior citizen with nagging arthritis, she doesn't venture as far afield in the office as she used to, spending much of her time in the ward with the boarding cats, looking out the window at the bird feeder.

She is the employee in the office with the smallest paycheck, the best benefits package, and the second-longest tenure, and as such, she warrants a place of honor in the Seven Bends family. She also holds the record for the hospital mascot with the longest reign, having surpassed both her predecessors by many years. This longevity is testament to a more robust constitution than Cy's, and a psyche less fragile than Ditto's. Long live the queen!

THE BEE'S KNEES

If you had told me when I was twenty that at fifty I would be practicing companion-animal medicine rather than equine medicine, I would have laughed you out of the room. If you had followed that prediction with one that said I would have no horses of my own, there might have been physical violence.

At twenty, I harbored in my mind a pastoral image of the acreage I would own one day. It would have twenty, maybe thirty acres of partly wooded land with ten or twelve acres of open pastures surrounded by white rail fences, two of which would form a lane lined with pear trees down the middle of the property, leading to a spacious home. The house would be perched on a rise overlooking the pastures and be separated from them by an expanse of lush green lawn, free of dandelions and mowed in a pleasing pattern of parallel lines. A dignified but playful golden retriever would be sitting on the front porch under the reaching white pillars and would have ambled with flagging tail out to the car as you drove into the circular paved entry. Beside the house, in a covered portico, would be parked my blue Chevy Silverado with its heavy-duty suspension and a white veterinary box with an array of drawers and cubbies and refrigerators filled with medications and supplies to treat the horses that were my patients. It might also contain a few doses of distemper vaccine to pop into the farm dogs, which would be the only canine patients I treated.

This image was so well developed in my mind at the time that I could not envision even one component of that scenario being different in my future. But, as you now well know, that picture does not describe my life in any way. What, you may ask, made the difference between my projected plan and my current reality? I can answer that question with two simple responses.

First, there was a sea change in my professional outlook. During my junior year in veterinary school, I was surprised to discover how much I enjoyed small-animal medicine. It provided me the opportunity to pursue what is most fun for me in veterinary medicine — the detective work of diagnosing diseases in patients that cannot tell you verbally where it hurts; the relative ease of working with animals that do not require a padded recovery room and a truck-size anesthesia machine; and the intensely sentimental aspects of companion-animal medicine, where decisions turn more on emotion than on economics.

These reasons were important in my decision, but to be honest, there was another dimension of horse practice that worried me. Please don't tell this to any horse people you may know; but at the time, I also realized that if I was to work on horses my whole life, I would have to deal with horse people. There is something unique about horse people that I am seldom confronted with in companion-animal practice. Every horse person knows everything about horses! Not only are all of them veritable horse whisperers, but they all want you to be fully aware of their equine genius. I know this to be true because when horses were my primary passion, it was with exactly this degree of respect that I regarded my own horse knowledge. I think this is coded on the same genes as a passion for horses.

To be fair, there are a few clients in small-animal practice that bring the same amount of self-taught knowledge to their interactions with their vet. Such people, though, account for only a small percentage of my clients. While typical pet owners do not come with this pride in their animal knowledge as standard equipment, horse people generally do, and it's a trait that I found tedious.

Add to that the fact that much in the horse world revolves around horse culture. This is true whether your equine focus is western pleasure, three-day eventing, dressage, hunter/jumper events, conformation showing, or racing. Around each of these subspecialties has developed a world in which the participants speak a language and follow a set of rules to which the rest of the world is simply not privy. Immersion in one of these cultures provides a certain translatable advantage in another. But lacking exposure, as I did, to all of these cultural climates was a handicap that made horse practice virtually unassailable for me — a handicap that I would have eventually tired of accommodating. Medicine is hard enough as it is.

That explains why I am a fulfilled companion-animal practitioner. But it does not explain why, at fifty, I still have no horses of my own. Simply stated, it's my kids' fault! I did try very hard to develop in Jace and Tucker a love for horses similar to that shared by Cynthia and me. We extolled the wonderful virtues of horses and regaled our sons with horse stories. I related with suitable embellishments the countless tales of my nine summers as a camper in Florida and the six summers I spent as a staff member in a horse barn. Cynthia added her memories of Mike and Ike, Tangerine, and the other horses she had growing up as a child in Tennessee. When they were old enough, we enrolled Jace and Tucker in summer horse camp, where they spent hours circling a ring at a somnolent walk on horses that wanted to go no faster. All our efforts, though, were to no avail. If the horse-loving genes are not present at birth, the passion apparently cannot be evoked by even the most creative of parental tactics.

The final nail was driven into the coffin of my horse-owning hopes on Jace's seventh birthday. We were camping at Camp Roosevelt in Fort Valley, the historic first of many Civilian Conservation Corps work camps in the 1930s where unemployed men were put to work planting trees, building roads, and keeping at bay the ravages of the Great Depression. You get to Camp Roosevelt by taking the Edinburg Gap Road east off Highway 11 on the north end of Edinburg and cresting the mountain at Tasker Ridge. As you descend into Fort Valley, you can stop partway down if you wish and fill a gallon jug or two with the fresh mountain rainwater that issues from springs and is dispensed through pipes by the roadway. You would think such water might carry a high risk of contamination when you look at the rudimentary delivery system that has been in place for generations. But you would be wrong; many families have used this free springwater as their main water supply for decades. If you turn south on Fort Valley Road at King's Crossing and follow the road to the apex of the valley, it eventually heads east and ascends over Edith Gap and down into the Page Valley, where Luray spreads out sleepily on the valley floor along the banks of the North Fork of the Shenandoah River. Just before you reach the top of Edith Gap, Camp Roosevelt is nestled into a couple of acres of sheltered woods and boasts ten camping spots that are claimed on a first-come, first-served basis and paid for on the honor system. Those campsites are filled with families in tents most summer weekends from Memorial Day to Labor Day.

On that beautiful April day, I had the brilliant idea of taking the family on a trail ride. There is a wonderful little stable in the Fort that has a warren of trails in the surrounding woods and a barn full of suitably calm trail horses. I had called a few days earlier and reserved four spots on the eleven o'clock ride on Jace's birthday. I thought this would be another chance to reinforce the ongoing horse indoctrination of the boys, and I was looking forward to it. During my six summers at camp, I had taken thousands of such rides, and even though I knew this one would be an hour of slow trudging, it would at least provide Jace and Tucker with another opportunity to feel the thrill of having the control of a thousand-pound beast in your hands, which had for me been intoxicating.

We arrived a half hour before our scheduled ride to let the boys walk up and down the line of tethered horses, whose tails lazily chased away the inevitable flies that pestered their sides and legs. Tucker was drawn to the big bay horse with the four white socks and the blaze of white streaking his forehead. The wrangler told us his name was Blaze and let Tucker stroke his nose and offer the carrots we had brought with us. Jace had difficulty choosing between a palomino mare named Queen and a buckskin gelding, creatively named Bucky, with a black mane and tail. His decision was made for him when the wrangler told us that the buckskin liked to trot on the trail rides. After that, Jace was all about Queen, offering stirring summaries of the exceptional virtues of mares and the many advantages that palominos offered over buckskins. Besides, he told us, Queen reminded him of the toy horse he had loved in kindergarten, which he had called King Horse.

When the time came to mount our horses, Jace was assisted onto the saddle of the palomino, where he immediately grasped the saddle horn and pasted an anxious look of concern on his now seven-year-old face. Tucker sat astride Blaze and surveyed the saddle and reins as a NASCAR fan would the dashboard of a race car, no doubt searching for the accelerator. This is Tucker's typical bring-it-on approach to a new activity. (I learned recently, as we were discussing the horse camp that we had placed such high hopes in, that Tucker had spent the entire two-week period wanting to, as he put it, "get the dang horse to run. How long can one person be expected to circle the ring at a walk anyway?" he asked.) It was with this same full-speed-ahead determination that Tucker turned his horse into the queue, his little legs barely reaching the stirrups, which were raised as high as possible.

Cynthia was put on Cheyenne, a staid and dependable black mare with a Roman nose and an apparent disregard for any cues a rider might give her. Cheyenne was committed to one simple goal — getting back to the stable after having expended as little energy as possible. That meant, apparently, following the horse ahead of her by matching each of its steps with a plodding one of her own, head down and eyes partially closed. Reins, stirrups, voice and weight commands, even the firm clumping of Cynthia's heels on Cheyenne's sides were all so many unnecessary and extraneous annoyances to the single-minded mare. All that she needed for navigational purposes was provided by the rump of the horse ahead of her.

Having been sure to make the wrangler well aware of my prodigious skills and limitless experience with horses of this sort, I was placed on a horse that required more in the way of direction than did Cheyenne. Bingo was a six-year-old paint gelding with, as I was assured by the wrangler, a little bit of "spirit" in him. I expected this meant I would need to be constantly vigilant to avoid losing control of a headstrong horse with a big heart and a will to run. To the wrangler, though, "spirit" apparently had a more biblical meaning: that Bingo possessed the "breath of life." In actual fact, it meant that the wrangler expected Bingo to remain awake for the duration of the ride. At least that's what seemed to be occurring as we left the paddock, where the horses had been loosely tied to the top rail of the fence.

Still, with Cynthia just ahead of Jace's horse and me just ahead of Tucker's, we headed out with high spirits, both Cynthia and I barking instructions at the boys and keeping up a steady stream of verbal encouragement. There were, as I recall, six or eight other guests whom the sole wrangler leading the trail ride was responsible for. I remembered from my years leading trail rides how it felt to have the safety of novices in my hands, and I felt good that Cynthia's valuable horse experience and mine could so drastically reduce his stress level, freeing him to concentrate on the other riders in the group, who, no doubt, needed more supervision. The line of horses headed into the woods, following a trail that the horses had taken hundreds of times before.

As the ride progressed, I could see that the lines of stress on Jace's face were easing as Cynthia's dialogue continued. His confidence was growing, and his mastery of his mount was having the desired effect as we wound through the trees and up the gentle hills. From my conversation with Tucker, I could tell that he was having fun, too. Both were, I was sure, beginning to experience the wonder and majesty of horsemanship. I began to picture in my mind the time when, as a family, we would head out on trail rides on horses of our own, perhaps packing camping gear behind our saddles for weekend pack trips in the mountains. Cynthia kept turning in her saddle to give me an encouraging look and a furtive thumbs-up. We were doing well!

It was at about the halfway point, where the trail turned into a particularly thick section of woods, that my horse-owning visions came to an abrupt and unexpected end. The four of us were at the tail end of the line of horses that entered that wood. It was the first horse or two in the line that initially disturbed the underground nest of hornets. Upon the initial equine invasion, two or three hornet scouts were dispatched to assess the enemy. They circled the line of horses and returned to the nest to alert the awaiting battalions that an attack on the invaders was necessary. By the time the full brunt of the assault was mounted by the indignant hornets, only the last four horses in the line were still in disputed territory. It was at these horses that the ten or twelve thousand buzzing fighters directed their fury — those and the hapless people who were riding them, unaware of the catastrophe that was about to be unleashed.

My first indication that something was amiss was when Cheyenne veered sharply from the trail and picked up speed, attempting to brush the stinging hornets off on the underbrush that whisked past with ever-increasing velocity. This, unfortunately, did not stop the onslaught, so she lunged, headlong and bucking, and circled back around. I looked up to see Cynthia and Cheyenne bearing down on us at full speed from the right of the path. Still at a full canter, she crossed in front of me and headed into the woods to my left. Just as Cynthia's cues to Cheyenne when she wanted her to speed up were ignored, so were her frantic attempts at slowing the horse now as it blazed new and exciting trails through the thick undergrowth. Finally, through superhuman effort and sheer force of will, Cynthia brought Cheyenne to a halt in the middle of the thick woods, the mare standing stock-still with feet planted, sweating and quivering in utter fear and confusion.

The sudden disappearance of Cheyenne from the line left an unexpected gap in front of Queen, who clearly felt it a mistake in need of immediate correction. Her impetus to do so was increased exponentially by the sudden and simultaneous attachment of two angry hornets: one to the soft skin on her muzzle and the other to a spot just above her tail. This so surprised her that she ran to the unwitting horse in front of her and immediately plunged her hurting nose into its unsuspecting fanny, then commenced rubbing her nose vigorously on the horse's rump. Apparently, this is considered among horses to be an incredibly rude gesture requiring a firm response. The horse immediately lashed out at Queen, landing a poorly aimed kick squarely on Jace's shin.

I watched with horror as the look on Jace's face turned from engaged and eager to sheer terror in less time than it takes to tell. Time slowed to stop-motion as with dread I watched three or four more hornets begin to hone in on Queen's neck, sides, and legs. I knew that within just a few seconds, she would erupt like a barrel of Prohibition moonshine. This would be more than Jace could tolerate. An intervention was obviously necessary, so I spurred Bingo firmly in the ribs with my heels, trying to close the distance between our horses. My plan was to reach down, grab the leather reins that Jace had let slip to the ground, and lead Queen to safety. Unfortunately, I had not adequately prepared Bingo for such an act of heroism. Just as I leaned down and reached for her reins, Bingo fell victim to a cowardly but effective hornet attack on his fanny. He wheeled around in the opposite direction from where I was heading and neatly deposited me in a pile at Queen's feet. Instinctively, and quite bravely, I might add, I reached up and grabbed the end of the reins that still dangled from her bit. In the same instant, Queen recoiled from the writhing human that had suddenly material-ized at her feet, rearing back and flailing with her front feet, striking fear into my core. I looked up to see Jace huddled over the saddle horn, hanging on gamely with both hands, his face white and streaked with fear. I realized that continuing to hold on to the reins would be good for neither Jace nor me, and I let go just in time for a hornet to plunge his stinger into my wrist with ma-levolent vengeance.

It was at about this time that Cheyenne's temporary paralysis disappeared, most likely cured by another hornet sting, and she erupted again into a headlong rush, Cynthia clinging to her as she ran under branches too low to be ducked, leaving long scratches that oozed parallel stripes of blood on Cynthia's cheeks and arms. As Cheyenne ran by me, I stood and spread my arms in an attempt to snag her bridle. This caused her to shy sharply to her right, a move for which Cynthia was unprepared. It was only by an amazing feat of horsemanship that she was able to remain in place on her saddle and once again gain control of Cheyenne just in time to avoid a wild race to the barn.

Despite all the excitement, Blaze plodded along the trail with Tucker on board, completely unperturbed by either the rodeos breaking out around him or the threat of the hornets that buzzed by his ears. When he reached the line of horses that had stopped on the trail, their riders watching the scene play out like rubberneckers at a highway pileup, Blaze simply stopped, chocked a rear toe up on the ground, and hung his head in boredom.

Cheyenne's second outbreak forced Queen back toward the end of the line of waiting horses, where I was now standing. I grabbed her bridle and she calmed noticeably and started rubbing her nose on my arm. Strangely, at this point some signal was sent to the squadrons of hornets to abandon the attack, and they disappeared as quickly as they had come. When it was over, I had been stung a total of four times: once on the wrist, once on the neck, and once on each knee.

The wrangler finally made his way around the waiting line of horses to where the Coston family had gathered at the end of the line. He found me on the ground, holding the bridle of Jace's mount. Cynthia was gamely steadying Cheyenne's nerves. The mare was lathered and frantic, fairly cantering in place. Tucker was surveying with envy the excitement of the rest of the family, seated astride Blaze, whom I'm sure I heard snoring. And Bingo was grazing luxuriously on the grass that grew some forty yards away from the trail, his saddle askew, one stirrup squarely on his back and the other hanging from his belly like the pendulum of a grandfather clock. The wrangler stopped, took in the scene, and then turned a stony gaze on me as I stood before him, rubbing the places on my wrist that had begun to swell and turn red.

"Hornets," I stammered by way of explanation.

But I don't think he believed me. I doubt he even heard me, since he had already turned his horse to retrieve Bingo. It seemed to take an inordinate amount of time, with me standing self-consciously in front of the group, for him to readjust Bingo's saddle so I could once again mount up. The other riders seemed put out that their ride had been interrupted. I think it was just coincidence that made the wrangler position me directly behind his horse for the return trip to the barn. From there, I could barely see Jace or Tucker or Cynthia at the end of the line.

By the time we made it back to the barn, the pain from my hornet stings had begun to ease, though the agony of my throbbing ego still smarted. To add insult to injury, it was many days before my fanny had recovered enough so that sitting on it was bearable again. I'm quite sure that was the last time I rode a horse. Since that day, there have been no forces in heaven or on earth that have ever been able to dredge up in Tucker or Jace even the slightest shred of equine interest. Their fancies have turned to water skiing and snow skiing, sports that, as a consequence, have taken on much more importance for Cynthia and me.

It's really not fair, I suppose, to place the blame for my lost dream on the boys. After all, both of them are away at college now. Cynthia and I could certainly take up our old hobbies once again if we chose to. It's funny, though, how time alters childhood dreams, how what was a joy to me when I was young now seems simply another chore that would take me away from the familiar comforts of routine. Perhaps it's the creeping advance of age and the betrayal of youthful priorities. But I don't think so. That would diminish the value of experience and the accumulated wisdom of maturity and would ignore the evolution of personal development.

The truth is, I am not the same person I was when I was twenty. Life has changed me. Marriage, fatherhood, and a career devoted to significant effort have ennobled, not eroded, me. I have not turned my back on previous passions. I have had new passions open before me. Is this not the stuff of life? Isn't this evolving self the spice that keeps life interesting and progressive? So celebrate with me the passions of youth. Relive them with nostalgia; recall them with humor. Then turn and allow new ones to overtake you. At fifty, with shoulders now sore from this season's first slalom run behind our boat, I have found this to be a wise course of action for me. It's also much easier on my bum. Come to think of it, I haven't been stung on the knee by a hornet since Jace's seventh birthday.

My Run-in with the Law

I happened to be standing in the lobby of the hospital one afternoon as a state trooper drove up the driveway in his cruiser. I watched with curiosity as Trooper Dalkins unfolded his six-foot-three-inch frame from the driver's seat of the car.

Trooper Dalkins had been a client of mine for many years. I had watched his two basset hounds grow from rambunctious adolescents to noble geriatric patients during that time. My mind flooded with the memory of the infected growth on Beau's front leg, which had responded miraculously to antibiotics after I had assured him and his wife that it would not. Then the scene replayed in my mind of Trooper Dalkins, his wife, and three daughters gathered around the examination table on which Beau lay, too ill to lift his head, before I slipped the medication into his vein that would ease him from his intractable and untreatable illness. It had been a touching and utterly excruciating scene, the tearful good-bye a loving family had bestowed upon a faithful friend after many years of devotion. I liked the Dalkins family very much.

When I had posed the most inappropriate of questions, Trooper Dalkins had answered it without comment or complaint. I suppose I am not the only one who has asked a state trooper the question. He was probably accustomed to it.

"How fast can I really drive on the interstate without one of you guys pulling me over?"

He had laughed offhandedly and told me that it was generally safe to go about six to eight miles per hour faster than the sixty-five limit posted on the highway signs.

"Yeah, if you go any faster than seventy-four, the troopers are going to start paying attention. But slower, you're generally going to be okay."

It had been several years since I had posed that question to Trooper Dalkins. But every time I drove past a cruiser hidden behind a knoll in the median of Interstate 81 at seventy-two or seventy-three miles per hour, I thought of him, grateful for the insider information he had provided. Armed with that information, I had not been pulled over on the highway since college days.

I was pleased to see Trooper Dalkins that day, since it had been a couple of years since Beau, his last pet, had passed away. We shot the breeze nonchalantly over the reception desk for a few minutes.

"Hey, you guys need to clamp down on the truckers on the highway a little tighter," I said to him. "Just yesterday, one of them literally pushed me off I-81 at full speed. He just came over into my lane without a thought. I had to swerve onto the grass to avoid him. That was exciting at seventy miles an hour."

"Yeah, it can get a little dicey out there, for sure." He leaned heavily on his elbow on the desktop, his biceps bulging his sleeve. The sidearm and his sheer bulk would be intimidating to any lawbreakers on the highway. He paused for a moment before asking, "So, what kind of car are you driving now?"

"It's just a little Nissan Maxima," I responded. "Not much of a car compared to those big eighteen-wheelers."

"That's for sure. You gotta drive defensively." Another pause. "What year is your car?"

I'm not much of a car guy; I am equipped with very little car pride. I'm happy if my vehicle just gets me to where I'm going. Details like engine size, available features, or even the model year don't stay with me for long. I searched my memory for this bit of trivia.

"Runs in my mind it's a 2003 or 2004, something like that."

"So it's one of the newer body styles, huh?"

"Yeah, I guess so."

He nodded his head lazily as he scanned the few people seated in the lobby, awaiting their turn to be called into the exam rooms with their pets. Then he turned to me again. "So, what color is your car?"

The question seemed a little strange to me at the time. He must be a car junkie, I thought, unlike me. Or perhaps he was still trying to imagine how a trucker could have missed seeing me and driven me off the road.

"It's gray, so I guess a trucker could have missed it in the evening light. But I honked and flashed my lights at him, and he just kept coming over."

Our conversation was interrupted by a page over the PA system, calling me to the treatment room to check on a patient. I waved good-bye to Trooper Dalkins and headed to the back to tend to my patient.

The case that awaited me soon erased the mounting confusion about the interaction with Trooper Dalkins, which had begun to tickle at the edges of my consciousness. A young sheltie had had a brush with a car and had suffered a fractured leg. The bone would need surgical repair, a procedure that was scheduled for the next day.

My mind was thoroughly occupied with planning the details of the surgery as I drove to work the next morning, that and appreciating the beauty of the spring on the mountains. The slopes were dotted with speckles of light purple where the redbud trees were blooming among the brilliant green of the budding oaks and the darker green of the mountain laurel. My mind wandered from the road. I had been on I-81 for only a few miles, driving absentmindedly in the passing lane, when I passed a state trooper's cruiser in the median. My eyes dropped like stones from the road down to my speedometer. Once again, I was relieved to see that I had set my cruise control at seventy-two miles an hour. Trooper Dalkins had saved me again!

Out of idle curiosity and without the slightest concern, I looked into my mirror. I was mildly surprised to see the cruiser nosing into traffic behind me. A rush of adrena-

line flooded my veins, my heart rate acceler-
ated involuntarily, and I slowed the car
down. This is silly, I reminded myself.
Trooper Dalkins's advice had always served
me well. I took a few deep breaths to calm
my nerves. Certainly, this trooper was after
someone else. But a quick scan of my mir-
rors failed to show any other drivers but the
one I had just passed. Must be an accident
ahead, I thought. But the needle on my
internal stress meter spiked again as I
watched the cruiser pull in behind me and
flip on his blue lights.

I was immediately assaulted by two separate but equally disturbing thoughts, which
attacked me like tag-team wrestlers, fast and
violently. The first was a quiet curse on
Trooper Dalkins. He had failed me! Though
his warnings had proved true for many
years, they had finally left me unprotected.
I had set the cruise control at seventy-two,
just as he had suggested, and yet here I was
being dragged to the side of the road by
these blasted blue lights. Trooper Dalkins,
I'm going to get you for this!

The second thought was that I was going
to have to call Jim at the school transporta-
tion department. For a couple of years, I
had been a volunteer bus driver at my sons'
school, logging countless hours behind the

wheel of the forty-nine-person coach, driving for music trips, varsity games, and a variety of other school functions. It was a ready excuse for being present at most of my children's school events and made me feel good about volunteering my time. It was also just plain fun to drive the big rigs. I had driven the coach through New York City on more than one occasion, even parallel-parking it once beside St. Patrick's Cathedral. Getting a ticket would mean that I would have to inform Jim of my infraction. That would be embarrassing at the very least and might reduce the amount of driving I would be allowed to do — not a thought I relished.

With these thoughts swirling in my mind, I watched in my rearview mirror as the officer approached my car, half-hoping that the man in uniform would be Trooper Dalkins. But as the officer reached the car and leaned down to look in the window, I realized with regret that I did not recognize him.

"Do you know why I pulled you over?"

"I'm guessing it's because I was going a bit too fast."

"Yes, sir, you were. I clocked you at seventy-five miles per hour."

I thought about pointing out that his radar couldn't possibly be right, since I had set the cruise control at seventy-two. But honestly, it seemed a silly argument to make.

"That's a little faster than I thought I was going."

"Is there a reason you were speeding?"

This seemed like a ridiculous question to me. There were, of course, a million reasons why I was speeding: I had gotten up a bit late and was running behind; I had gotten behind a school bus, which had slowed me down even more; there were important things waiting for me at the office; I had grown up in a family of habitual speeders and was a victim of my genetic heritage; my car had tempted me to take advantage of its pep. I could have tried to play the trump card and claim there was a life-and-death emergency waiting for me at the office. But honestly, none of my justifications seemed valid as I looked at the gun holstered at the officer's side.

"Not any reasons that would make sense to you, sir," I responded weakly, resigned to my punishment.

"In that case, I'm going to have to issue you a citation for driving in excess of the speed limit." His words sounded officious and punitive, like a judgment of the court. "If you'll give me your license and registration, I'll go back to my cruiser and write up

218

the citation."

The time it took him to go back to his car and write that ticket seemed an eternity. I watched him furtively in the mirror, drumming my fingers on the dashboard and shaking my head in frustration. I was sure that in a small community like mine, the drivers of every car that passed recognized me. It struck me as I sat there that my name and my crime would be printed in the community section of the weekly newspaper for all to see. No doubt, my lead foot would be the topic of discussion around many supper tables in the days to come.

"Did you hear that the vet got a ticket for speeding the other day?" my clients would say to one another. "What a shame. You'd think you could count on your veterinarian to obey the laws, wouldn't you? What is this world coming to?" I envisioned my loyal clients during their appointments in the days ahead, clucking their tongues and shaking their heads at me in reproach, disappointed and disgusted at my lawlessness.

Finally, I saw the car door open and the officer emerge from his cruiser carrying a sheaf of paperwork. He pushed an important-looking form through my window on a clipboard. I knew it was the ticket I deserved.

"You are being cited for going seventy-five miles per hour in a sixty-five-mile-an-hour zone. You are to appear in Shenandoah County General District Court in three weeks to answer this charge."

"If I want to just pay the fine, do I still have to appear in court?"

"No, sir, you can go to the clerk's office and pay the fine if you do not wish to defend yourself. If you do that, this offense will appear on your permanent record and will be reflected in your insurance rates."

"Yes, I'm sure they will. Does that mean they won't if I show up at court?" I asked.

"They will if you are found guilty of the crime."

"But there's hardly any chance I will be found innocent, is there?"

"I did clock you at seventy-five, sir."

"Yes, that's what you said."

"Do you have any other questions?"

What is there to have questions about? I wondered. I had been caught red-handed, having trusted the word of a state trooper. I wouldn't make that mistake again. It had cost me a stiff fine, the privilege of being a volunteer bus driver, and would undoubtedly jack up my insurance rates.

"I don't think so."

"Okay, if there are no other questions, please sign the citation on the line I have marked with an *X*," the officer continued, tapping the clipboard with his pen on the line where I was to sign.

I took his pen and quickly signed my name in the space provided. But when I tried to hand the clipboard to the officer, he pushed it back toward me roughly.

"In order to make sure we have made everything clear to you, please read the information on the next page, as well."

I looked up at him with confusion on my face. I had been in college the last time I had received a speeding ticket, but I didn't recall any additional information. Perhaps law enforcement was trying to be more consumer-friendly these days, but something about the officer's approach and carriage made me question whether customer service was his number-one priority. He was pointing at the clipboard, a stern look on his face.

I flipped the citation over, looking for the additional information he had mentioned. I found only a sheet of yellow notebook paper on which some words had been quickly scrawled in a familiar script. This made no sense at all. I held the clipboard closer so I could read the words. "APRIL FOOLS',

DOC! GOTCHA AGAIN!" And in smaller letters below: "Don't be mad. You know we love you. Your family at Seven Bends (excluding Susan, Diane, and Marti)."

Quickly I read the words again, my mind spinning. My head jerked up to the trooper's face. He was laughing now. I watched the gun in his holster jiggle with his mirth. He had his cap off and was wiping his eyes with the back of his hand.

"You dog!" I said, smiling now myself. "Who put you up to this?"

The officer was laughing too hard to answer. In reply, he simply pulled his fist up, his thumb pointing behind my car. I looked in my rearview mirror, surprised to find that now there were two state trooper cruisers parked behind me, both of their racks of lights spinning blue. Walking up behind the officer who had pulled me over was another man in uniform, who was also laughing uproariously. I recognized Trooper Dalkins right away! He was laughing too hard to speak.

"So that's why you were in my office yesterday!"

He nodded his head weakly, the effort of trying to answer me apparently too much for him.

"And that's why you wanted all that

information about my car, too! I can't believe you got roped into this." That's when the lightbulb went on in my dimly lit brain. "This was all Rachel's doing, wasn't it?"

The two officers of the law were now leaning on each other's shoulders and holding their sides. Finally, Trooper Dalkins gathered himself enough to meet my gaze. But he just shrugged and kept smiling, coconspirator to the end.

"So, I'm really not getting a ticket after all?" I asked incredulously.

Trooper Dalkins and his cohort simply shook their heads, unable to quit laughing.

"I don't have to show up in court, either?" I said, more to myself than to the two helpless officers. They couldn't hear me anyway, given their ongoing laughter.

Those two state troopers were still laughing as I pulled away from their parked cruisers; their lights and their grins were still flashing. But I was laughing, too. Sometimes there is nothing to do but enjoy it when you are the butt of such a stunt. Rachel was proving herself to be a worthy adversary.

When I got to the office, I put on a stern face of feigned anger and stormed into the lobby. I marched past the reception desk without a greeting and went immediately to the staff break room, where I tacked the summons up on the bulletin board. I scrawled one sentence across the bottom of the ticket in large red letters: "You're all fired — excluding Susan, Diane, and Marti." But it was weak retaliation. Once again, I had been had! April Fools' indeed!

BRANSON MISERY

The phone was clamoring for attention the moment I walked into the house that Sunday evening. Somehow I had a bad feeling about it. As a solo practitioner, I had learned to fear the ringing of the phone. So often it meant that I would miss supper with the family or be called away from my children's school program or have to leave the lawn half-mowed.

When I heard Mrs. Kovac's voice on the other end of the line, my apprehension eased a bit. I didn't mind so much being interrupted when the ones needing help were some of my favorite clients. Local merchants, Mrs. Kovac and her husband were regular visitors with their forty-pound beagle, Branson. You really couldn't help liking the Kovacs. Ever courteous and gracious, they were pillars of the community. Both spoke in quiet, relaxed tones, seldom raising their voices. Neither was excitable

225

beyond the quick and easy chuckle that epitomized their approach to life.

Their devotion to Branson, who was in many respects their polar opposite, was undeniable and obvious. Since their children had long since left home, Branson willingly accepted his status as most favored dependent in the Kovac home.

Granted, Branson did need special attention. That much was true. For years, he had fought chronic ear problems, which had thickened the skin on his pendulous ears and required the Kovacs to clean his ears daily and apply medications even more often than that. As beagles are prone to do, Branson had also developed thyroid problems, which made him plump, to be kind, and required supplementation with pills twice daily. He also battled bouts of skin allergies, which sent him into paroxysms of intense itching, reddened his skin, and predisposed him to recurrent infections on his tummy and legs. All of these problems made Branson a frequent visitor at the hospital.

We always had advance warning that he was coming, since Branson displayed another common beagle trait. As soon as the Kovacs put him in the car, he commenced to baying, a term that perfectly conveys the action, even if you have never heard the word. This mournful tune could be heard faintly at first, then more loudly, as the Kovacs' car neared the clinic. It reached an earsplitting crescendo as they eased into a parking space in front of the office. Listening to the racket, you expected to look out the window and find a pack of hunting dogs surrounding a treed raccoon. Instead, you just saw Branson in the backseat, his nose and tail pointed skyward, howling in full cry, with the Kovacs in the front seat, courtly and proper as always, stoically suffering the cacophany with taut, strained faces. Branson's baying would continue as he lunged eagerly toward the door of the office, snapping the leash tight and pulling Mr. Kovac along like a water-skier.

Examinations and consultations were generally completed amid this din, which required that all conversation be conducted in uncharacteristically loud voices to override Branson's joyous celebration of having completed his physical and being put down on the floor again. Branson's whole life seemed to be spent in unreserved and verbal anticipation of the amazing excitement that lay just ahead.

But this night was different. Branson was not his usual overexuberant self. He was sick! For two hours, he had been vomiting continuously. Mrs. Kovac had waited to call me, though, till Branson vomited up a large amount of bright red blood. This frightened her — and rightly so. It frightened me, too!

"I think you should bring him over right away," I said when she called.

Upon his arrival, I knew instantly that something was terribly wrong with Branson. His head was down and he was struggling for breath. He was slobbering excessively and choking on the thick saliva that trailed from the corners of his mouth. He seemed too tired to stand and, at the same time, too uncomfortable to lie down. Mrs. Kovac, expecting the worst, had been too emotional to come. Despite his concern, though, her husband maintained his calm, quiet bearing.

"Branson's really under the weather this time, Dr. Coston. I can't imagine what got all this started. He was fine earlier in the day."

"You say he vomited some blood?" I asked.

"Oh my, yes, a whole lot of blood. I can't believe he could lose that much without it affecting him."

"Oh, he's affected all right, Mr. Kovac. Look how pale his gums are," I said as I pulled up Branson's lips. They were pasty and white, with hardly any visible pink.

"I just knew he was in real trouble. What do you think is going on?"

"He's got to have a bleeding ulcer in his stomach for him to lose that much blood. But the question is, Why?"

My mind fumbled for the possible causes of bleeding in the stomach. Regardless of the inciting cause, the bleeding had to be stopped right away.

"Mr. Kovac, this is a serious condition and it needs to be treated quickly. I'll need your help."

With Mr. Kovac acting as assistant, I placed an intravenous catheter, started fluid administration, and drew some blood for testing. Mr. Kovac was then dispatched to the corner convenience store for a bag of ice. While he was gone, I anesthetized Branson and placed him on his stomach on the surgical table. After giving him antacids, medication for shock, and antibiotics, I looked over the results of the blood tests. Things were not looking good for the home team. Branson had lost a lot of blood; his red-cell count had dropped to half of what it should have been.

Mr. Kovac returned and I began to flood Branson's stomach with ice-cold water laced with epinephrine, a medication I hoped would shrink the size of the vessels. My hope was to stop the bleeding by constricting the vessels in the stomach with the medicine and the cold shock. A simple plan, perhaps, but my only hope, I thought. I knew that in his present condition, Branson would certainly not survive an operation, and that was the only other way I knew to stop the bleeding.

The next two hours were spent repeatedly filling Branson's stomach with the ice water, then draining it out again with a large tube. Little by little, the returning fluid became progressively less red, till finally there was no sign of blood. The crisis was averted, but we were no closer to answering the question of why the bleeding had started. Once stabilized, Branson would still need surgery. But that would have to wait a day or two, until his condition improved.

The next morning I dragged myself, tired and deflated, to the clinic with a feeling of dread. The night had been long and the rest had been short. But more than anything, I feared what I might find. In those days, before there was an emergency hospital staffed throughout the night with veterinarians and technicians, we were left with no options but to leave critically ill patients unattended in the hospital overnight. The following morning I might come in and find a patient either improved or deceased. I wasn't sure which situation I might find in Branson's cage that morning. It wasn't good. During the night, Branson had vomited again. The anxious look was back in his eyes and flecks of clotted blood speckled the bottom of the cage. His gums were just as white as before. Feeling defeated, I lifted the phone and called the Kovacs' home. Mr. Kovac answered.

"Things are really no better, I'm afraid."

I hate this part of the job perhaps more than any other. Not every patient can be saved, despite all our efforts. I know this intellectually and am reminded of it often enough, but each time the emotional sting is still intense.

"I think we need to make some decisions. Can you and your wife come over this morning as soon as possible?"

In the meantime, I took some X-rays and could just detect what looked like a small nodule in the wall of the stomach. Things began to make sense. My suspicion was that Branson had a tumor in his stomach that was producing a hormone that damaged his stomach's protective lining and increased the acid secretion in the stomach. Over time, the increase in acid had created ulcers, which had bled profusely. I was speculating, of course. Only surgery would confirm my suspicions, and I was sure Branson could not withstand such an invasive procedure. In the examination room, I faced the Kovacs with a heavy heart.

"Things are not looking good for Branson. I think he has a tumor in the lining of his stomach that is bleeding. It may be causing other ulcers, as well. I can't know this for sure without doing surgery to see if I can remove the tumor and stop the bleeding. The problem is, all the blood loss has left him weak and very compromised. I'm not sure his chances of pulling through even with surgery are very good. But without it, his odds are even worse."

Mrs. Kovac stood stock-still, her back straight as I spoke. But her eyes didn't once meet mine and her chin quivered with emotion. Mr. Kovac stooped slightly, his hands clasped behind his back. Each avoided the gaze of the other. The room was quiet for a long time. Then Mr. Kovac spoke in his quiet, measured way, this time punctuated by frequent emotional quavers.

"Dr. Coston, Branson's been a better friend than most any dog we've ever had. Better than a lot of people we've known, too. He's been even-tempered and loyal. He's been with us at home and kept us company at the office. He helped us raise our boys and comforted us when they left home. Even though we've had to doctor those ears and his skin all these years, it's never been a moment's bother to us 'cause we love him so much."

Mrs. Kovac's eyes never left the spot she had been studying on the tabletop. She was now rocking slowly from toe to heel and back again, the hem of her skirt swaying with the motion. She remained silent, her emotions just barely under control. I couldn't help noticing a tear drop from her cheek and land on the table as her husband continued his eulogy. She saw the splash as it landed and directed her gaze to the spot of wetness, but otherwise she did not respond to his words.

"You know, Dr. Coston, how much we love him and how much we have done for him in the past. And you know that if we thought he could recover, there is nothing we wouldn't do for him now."

Not trusting my voice, I nodded a reply before he continued, which he did after searching my face for any hint of hope or optimism. I could muster none, so I avoided

his eyes. He sighed deeply before continuing.

"But I know that part of loving him is being willing to say good-bye, too. Branson is
almost fifteen years old and he's lived every
minute of those fifteen years at full bore.
He wouldn't understand it if he had to be
throttled down now. Marion and I discussed
it on the way over here and I think we're in
agreement on this. We just cannot justify
continuing a hopeless fight, especially if his
chances are poor either way."

He paused briefly and glanced at his wife.
She nodded her head resolutely but otherwise didn't move.

"Branson has been a gentleman all his life.
He doesn't owe us anything. But we owe
him something now. We owe him the right
to say good-bye with dignity and not endure
a hopeless struggle just to preserve our selfish emotions."

There was a pause while all three of us
gathered ourselves. Then he continued.

"So we'd be obliged if you'd allow us to
be with Branson as you help him along.
Would you do that?"

I choked a too-brusque response and fled
the room to collect the medication. Through
bleary eyes I drew the solution into the
syringe, knowing that what would come

next would be torture for the Kovacs but release for Branson. Back in the room, I summarized the procedure for the Kovacs so that they would know just what to expect. Then I slipped the needle into the hub of the catheter and squeezed the plunger on the syringe, sending the blue solution into Branson's vein. His strained and anxious eyes relaxed for a brief moment before the spark of life left them. The muscles of his hard, tense abdomen eased their grip of pain. I knew Branson's suffering, pain, and discomfort were finally over. But the knowing didn't change the burden of loss and sadness.

The Kovacs continued to lovingly caress Branson's coat and smooth the graying muzzle long after I listened to the rhythm of his heartbeat fade. As I left the room, with those two lovely people bent over the still form of their noble friend, I heard Mr. Kovac in his quiet, now-choked voice whisper his last thoughts to his dog.

"Thanks, Branson. You've been quite a friend."

An hour later, after I had somewhat regained my composure and the Kovacs had paid their final respects, I picked up the record for my next patient and walked into the same room the Kovacs had vacated. This would be, I thought, a much-needed reprieve. Mrs. Allen was bringing her new puppy to see me for the first time. This would be a happier appointment than her last one. She had finally adopted a new puppy after losing an ancient shih tzu to cancer several months previously. I was eager to meet the new addition to the family.

But when I opened the door to the room, Mrs. Allen's eyes were brimming and red. I knew that sometimes the first visit after a traumatic loss can bring back painful memories. My first reaction was to reach around the exam table and give her a comforting hug. After she pulled away, somewhat embarrassed, she nodded to the whiteboard on the wall that I used to draw medical illustrations for my clients.

"That just brought back everything," she said by way of explanation.

I turned around and looked at the board. There in a faltering hand were written these words: "Thank you so much for understanding and caring. We loved Branson so much. The Kovacs."

THE COMPLACENCY OF ROUTINE

In the course of my practice, some things are done so frequently that they become routine. This is true, no doubt, in all professions. I suppose it is routine, for instance, for Tiger Woods to nonchalantly flip a golf ball out of a deep sand trap to within a few inches of the hole, or for Michael Jordan to fake a drive and instead put up a jump shot that hits nothing but net just at the buzzer. It is routine for Michael Phelps to slice with such speed through the water, pushing his body to shave off that extra hundredth of a second and set a new world record. For world-class athletes, their feats are routine because they have done them countless times before. For me, surgical sterilization is a routine task. I suppose I have performed many thousands of spays over the years. I could probably spay a dog or a cat in my sleep.

But the truth is that there is really no such

thing as a routine medical procedure. Each time I make a spay incision, I remind myself that, for this patient, it will probably be the most dramatic event of her life so far. What is routine for me is definitely not routine for my patients — or for their owners. The challenge with routine surgeries is to remember that at any moment it may become a complicated, life-threatening emergency. Consequently, I, must maintain meticulous attention to detail and strict adherence to correct protocol. Muffin was an example of just how quickly things can change.

Muffin was a twelve-year-old Yorkshire terrier owned by the Ardens, who doted on her altogether too much, though neither Muffin nor her owners would have admitted it. Mr. and Mrs. Arden were the quintessential American retirees. He was perhaps in his eighties when I first met him, of medium height, with puffy eyes and hair fixed into position with Brylcreem. He wore wire-rimmed glasses and polyester slacks. Generally, he was pleasant to deal with. His wife, a short, worried woman with bluish hair and a thin face, was a few years younger than her husband and had clearly left the details of life to him for decades. The pair had, unfortunately, lost a bit of their sharpness with age, usually breezing into the office with Muffin tucked into the crook of an arm. They seldom had an appointment, though they always distinctly remembered having made one.

Their befuddled approach extended to Muffin's health as well, making her preventive care a bit haphazard and their office visits challenging. I learned, for instance, that trying to garner a history from them was an impossible task, as they would invariably veer sharply away from my question to subjects far afield from the topic at hand. To their confusion was added a significant degree of hearing loss — his worse than hers — which was accentuated by the shrill whistled duet of their hearing aids. Until I figured these things out, conversations with them about Muffin's issues toggled between confusing and downright amusing.

"So, have you had any health concerns with Muffin since I last saw her?" I would ask innocently.

Mrs. Arden would look at me, confused, then begin fiddling with the volume on her hearing aid. With utmost confidence, Mr. Arden would fix me with a benevolent smile and say something like "You, too! Thanks for the compliment." Then he would slap me good-naturedly on the shoulder, chuckling.

"Jim, I think he was asking about Muffin," Mrs. Arden would bay, pointing repeatedly at the little dog in his arms.

"Yes, Lovey, that's why we're here." And then they would both look at me expectantly, smiling sweetly.

I'd try again at higher decibel levels. "So has everything been going okay with Muffin?"

"Oh yes, yes," he'd respond, "without any trouble at all. And almost every day for the last two or three weeks."

"Almost every day, what?"

"What's that you say?"

"You said she had done it almost every day. Done what?"

"Sure has!" he'd reply. "But that's no different from before. She's always done that."

"Done what?"

And Mr. Arden would throw his head back and laugh appreciatively, like I had just told his favorite joke again. Who knows, maybe I had. Usually at some point during the appointment, they would get around to describing their concerns and I would be able to get across to them the most salient of Muffin's health-care instructions. Some days were definitely better than others.

I took to just looking at the record and administering whatever vaccines or tests were due, giving Muffin a thorough physical examination and prescribing any necessary medications. I always made sure the directions were clearly printed on the easy-to-open vials. This seemed to work best and always satisfied the Ardens, who would shake my hand appreciatively and trundle Muffin back into the car.

Though it was often unclear just how much of the information I gave them truly sank in, there was no doubt about how much they adored Muffin. They showed their devotion to her in the loving attention they paid her and the frequent visits to our office. In the many times I saw her, never did I see her feet hit the floor. Mr. Arden carried her everywhere, tucked like a purse into the crook of his arm.

It was a good thing Muffin was so loved, because she was one of those dogs with physical attributes that only doting parents could ignore. Since she so rarely walked on her own, she tended toward obesity, her stomach veritably dragging on the ground as she hobbled along. She also had problems with periodontal disease, which made her breath smell repulsive and had caused the loss of her lower canine teeth. Though this did not affect her ability to eat, it did prevent her from being able to contain her tongue, which lolled out of her mouth to one side in a most inebriated way. The large warts decorating her head and face and the cloudiness of age in her eyes added to the overall effect. To be kind, Muffin would not be up for any beauty awards — that much was certain.

One day the Ardens brought Muffin in for a routine teeth cleaning and the removal of the most offensive warts on her body. The planned procedure was nothing if not routine. I was not the slightest bit concerned, despite her advancing age. Admitting her that morning, I nonchalantly promised to take special care for her safety during the procedure and assured them I would call as soon as they could take their pet home that afternoon.

As I always do before anesthetizing my patients, I performed an examination of Muffin before administering the sedatives. Her eyes, ears, nose, and throat looked normal except for the age-related changes and the hard, dark tartar on her teeth. Her heart and lungs sounded fine when I listened to them with my stethoscope. I noted the location of the warts I would be removing as I examined the skin. Everything seemed in order. Then I felt Muffin's abdomen carefully. A large, smooth mass taking up a large proportion of the space in the abdomen was immediately apparent.

"Ooh boy," I said to Lisa. "Poor Muffin really has to urinate. Why don't you take her out and let her relieve herself before surgery?"

When Lisa returned after Muffin's potty break, I asked her if Muffin had urinated a large amount.

"Not really. She passed only a little bit. I expected more, from what you said, but no, she didn't have to go so bad after all."

I felt her stomach again. The lump was still there, as large as ever. A gnawing concern began to form in my brain. Carefully feeling the lump again, I tried to identify its borders and decipher exactly which organ was involved. My eyes closed and my forehead furrowed, I directed all my attention at what I was feeling with my fingers. All of a sudden I felt the mass give and suddenly change shape in my hand, like a miniature implosion.

I knew immediately what had happened. The tumor had burst! As often happens with rapidly growing masses, it had filled with blood and become exceedingly fragile. Though I was feeling it very gingerly, the capsule had broken like a balloon filled with Jell-O. I knew it was now bleeding unchecked into the abdomen.

Things really began to hop at that point. Muffin was taken directly into the X-ray room for abdominal X-rays. Her leg was shaved and prepped, an intravenous catheter was placed into her vein, and fluids were started. I instructed Lisa to take some blood for testing, then to start shock medications and sedatives in preparation for surgery. As she hurried to follow my instructions, I dialed the Ardens' number. They needed to know the seriousness of the situation. Mrs. Arden answered the phone.

"Hello, Mrs. Arden, this is Dr. Coston. In examining Muffin prior to surgery this morning, I discovered a mass in her abdomen. I'm afraid the mass has ruptured and I think she is bleeding internally."

There was a moment of silence on the other end of the phone. Then I heard Mrs. Arden chuckle quietly. "Yes, it is a nice day outside, isn't it?"

"Yes, it is," I replied. "But did you hear what I said about Muffin?"

"No, Muffin's not here. She's getting her teeth cleaned at Dr. Coston's office. He's such a kind doctor, don't you think?"

"This is Dr. Coston," I virtually yelled

into the phone.

"Oh, Dr. Coston. Is Muffin all right?"

"No, Mrs. Arden, she isn't. She has a tumor in her tummy that has burst and I need to take her to surgery right away."

I heard her speaking loudly to someone else in the room. I could hear the sudden strain and fear in her trembling voice.

"They have found a tumor in Muffin and she's not doing well. Oh, Jim, what are we going to do without her?"

I heard the phone change hands, and then Mr. Arden's voice came on the line, bright and full of courage and optimism. I was relieved to hear clear cognition in it that day, as well.

"My wife is all undone, Doctor. Tell me what you've found."

Quickly, I went over the findings of my physical examination and the current condition of his beloved companion, concerned that the details would not be fully understood. I heard an initial sigh of concern and resignation; then Mr. Arden's resolve returned.

"Okay, Doctor, do what you have to do. My wife and I will be right over. We'll just wait in the lobby for news. . . . And Dr. Coston, uh . . . what do you think the chances are?"

"At this point, I think they're about fifty-fifty. It could go either way, but we'll do our very best." I was glad that Mr. Arden was completely aware of the situation and its ramifications.

Within five minutes, the Ardens were waiting in the lobby. By this time, Muffin was anesthetized and being readied to go into the surgery suite. Quickly I poked my head into the waiting room and gave the Ardens some encouragement. Mrs. Arden put her head in her hands and sobbed. I had time only to offer a hug and a quick prayer before I had to leave them and attend to my patient.

In surgery, I found a large tumor attached to the spleen. As I had suspected, the tumor had burst and there was a large volume of blood pooling in the abdominal cavity, with more blood flowing freely from the fractured surface of the mass. As quickly as I could, I stopped the bleeding, then proceeded to remove the spleen.

With the spleen and the angry tumor in a bin, there was finally room for me to explore the rest of the abdominal organs. No other tumors were visible. With a sigh of relief, I flushed her belly with a liter or two of saline solution before suturing Muffin's abdomen closed. The procedure had taken about an hour and Muffin had held her own well. Now she just needed some time to recover.

I made my way down to the lounge, where the Ardens were waiting for me to finish my work. As I sat down beside them, drained from the unexpected stress of the morning, I noticed a woman I didn't recognized. Mrs. Arden, wringing her hands with anxiety, introduced us.

"Dr. Coston, this is our next-door neighbor, Ruth Madsen. When she heard about Muffin, she came over to sit with us. Everyone loves Miss Muffin, you know. How is she?"

"Muffin is doing well as of right now. The tumor involved about half of the spleen and had, as I feared, ruptured and was bleeding into the abdomen. It weighed almost a tenth of Muffin's body weight. We're fortunate! Had we waited even fifteen minutes more, I don't think she would have made it. But surgery went very well and I was able to get all of the tumor. She came through the surgery like a champ and is now in recovery. I think we're very fortunate to have a live patient at this point. Good thing she's a fighter."

"We're so grateful to you, Dr. Coston. So you think she's going to be okay?"

"Well, we're not completely out of the

woods yet, but we've done everything we can at this point. The rest is up to her. But I am optimistic. We do have to wait for the biopsy to come back before we can breathe easy, but a good percentage of these tumors are benign. If this one is, surgery will likely be curative. We're very lucky! As fragile as that tumor was, it was not a matter of if it was going to burst, but when."

"And I just bathed her yesterday. What if it had happened then?" Mrs. Arden was rightfully frightened.

"Fortunately, it didn't," I replied. "But if this had happened at home, she would never have survived it. It could easily have ruptured during a bath or when you were drying her. It could have happened just lifting her to take her outside. It was literally a time bomb waiting to explode."

During the next twelve hours, Muffin's recovery progressed well. Because she was tenuous that first night, I took Muffin home with me. She slept beside my bed, where I could check on her every hour. Our senior citizen kitty, Rush, ever the nursemaid, lay beside Muffin's bed and meowed each time she awoke. By morning, Muffin was much brighter, and I was confident that she would recover fully.

The Ardens were at the hospital bright

and early the next morning to check on their friend. Muffin greeted them excitedly.

"You wouldn't believe our neighbors, Dr. Coston. They were great. They took turns sitting with us all evening long. They even brought in supper for us. They were as concerned about Muffin as we were. She looks so much better this morning. She is going to be okay, isn't she?"

"Yes, I believe she is. If her progress continues at this rate, I expect to send her home to you this evening."

"When will we hear about the biopsy results?"

"I expect to hear in about five days. I'll call you as soon as I know anything."

Muffin did go home that night. In fact, with the tumor gone, her appetite and activity increased to levels well above what they had been for several months before the crisis. The biopsy came back benign, and Muffin lived several years after that fateful day.

I have thought of Muffin often since then, reliving the stomach-churning feeling of that tumor crumbling in my hand, the realization flooding me that what had begun as a mundane event had erupted in an instant into a full-throated emergency, thrusting a beloved life into the balance. It was a defining moment, one of many that separated me from my nonchalance and reminded me that few things in life are truly routine. Every trip to the grocery store, every interaction with friends, each moment of every day overflows with an abundance of promise, of adventure, of risk. An event, a life is routine only when we fail to appreciate its potential. Succumbing to the habit of experiencing everyday activities as drudgery or routine is simply too expensive a price to pay, for it sentences the whole of life to complacency. Embracing the excitement in the mundane, however, transforms each task into an adventure. Routine living occurs by default. Living life fully in the moment, fully alive, requires a conscious choice.

Muffin was no prettier after the surgery than before. Because of the turn of events, we did not get her teeth cleaned that day. Her tongue still hung out, her eyes were still shaded with age, and her face was still marred by warts. Because she felt so much better after the surgery and her devoted owners were that much less inclined to deny her anything, she became even a bit pudgier. She was, if anything, even less attractive to my eyes. But it was not my eyes that gazed at her with ever more unbridled affection. And it was the glint of that undaunted devotion so clearly evident in the wizened expressions on the faces of Mr. and Mrs. Arden as they looked at their old friend that was responsible for teaching me anew the lesson of immediacy.

When Muffin passed a year or two later, I thought that was the last I would see of the Ardens. But several weeks after her loss, they bumbled into the office one afternoon without an appointment, a tiny teacup Yorkie riding proudly in the crook of Mr. Arden's arm.

"What have you got there?" I asked, taking the tiny pup from him. The two of them beamed proudly at me as I fawned over the dog, which tipped the scales at barely two pounds.

"This is Muffin," Mr. Arden said, smiling broadly.

"No, Jim!" his wife corrected loudly. "Muffin died weeks ago, remember. This is Ginger!"

"Well, she is precious," I said, enchanted with the pup as she wiggled and licked at my earlobes. "Where did you find her?"

"She's about ten weeks old now, right, Lovey?" Mr. Arden's smiling face revealed no hint that he had answered some other question.

"No, not ten, darling," Mrs. Arden responded sweetly. "I think there were only four in the litter."

Ginger grew into a carbon copy of Muffin, even developing many of the same personality traits. Her feet saw the ground no more often than had her predecessor's, though she remained petite at four pounds. And the Ardens demonstrated the same unswerving devotion to her in her first years of life.

Then one day, she was brought in by a middle-aged couple I did not recognize. Jim Arden Jr. and his wife were taking her to their home in another state and had stopped by the office to pick up copies of her medical records. They told me that both of his parents had passed away within a week of each other. The memorial service for both of them had been held the day before in town. It was the last time I saw Ginger.

BUNNY DEMISE

Every year two events in our community bring a dramatic upsurge in the popularity of pet rabbits. The first is Easter, when advertisers feature cute bunnies dressed in pastel doll clothes that speak with cute cartoon voices and extol the virtues of a myriad of completely indispensable commodities. Those commercials pedal not only candy and toys and baby dolls; they also sell bunnies. Children seven years old and younger solicit from their doting parents those commodities, but they are especially insistent about the bunnies.

I can understand this desire. When I was a young boy growing up on Merritt Island in Florida, we drove past a house every day on South Tropical Trail that had a sign out front advertising RABBITS — DRESSED TO ORDER. For years, I dreamed of exactly how I wanted my pet bunny to be dressed. I waffled between a swashbuckling Robin

Hood outfit and a pastel blue Peter Rabbit costume. Either way, I knew my bunny would look beautiful. My folks, though, never gave in to my pleas for a costumed rabbit. It was only after years of incessant requests that they told me just what "Rabbits — Dressed to Order" meant. Imagine my horror!

The other event in our county that increases rabbit ownership is the annual Shenandoah County Fair. The County Fair is a big event in rural Virginia communities, drawing thousands to the midway and providing a common congregation point for the 4-H clubs and the farmers. When our boys were young, the Shenandoah County Fair was an opportunity for them to see every flavor of agriculture up close and personal. They saw pigs the size of small boats with litters of squealing piglets competing for one of the hugely engorged teats. They saw woolly lambs so young they teetered on spindly legs. They saw muscle-bound Charlois and Black Angus bulls so large that they towered over them, twice their height or more. Goats, chickens, pigeons, guinea pigs, rabbits, and even emus are all farmed in our county and make their annual appearance at the stock shows at the Shenandoah County Fair. Held around the week of Labor Day, it is the last summer bash before school starts again in early September.

Between the rides of the midway and the barns housing the livestock, you pass the rigged games of chance that heavily tattooed and chain-smoking roadie hooligans man, calling to you through bullhorns. Every year, at least one of these games gives away as prizes young rabbits. They are usually physiologically stressed to the max and come with no prior health care and are loaded with parasites inside and out.

At these two times of the year, parents across the county succumb to the pressure placed on them by their rabbit-coveting kids without giving much thought to the care these animals might need. Without proper nutrition, housing, or the slightest nod to appropriate rabbit husbandry, these families trail their ne'er-do-well bunnies through the offices of the county vets for weeks after Easter and the fair.

Rabbits can make wonderful pets when given adequate attention and training. I have rabbit patients who know their names, come when called, use litter boxes, and interact with the family in much the same way that cats or dogs do. They can be playful and mischievous and have wonderful, engaging personalities. They are solicitous of their owners' time and attention, following them around the house and lying down at their feet. They beg for food and treats, get spoiled and naughty, and wrestle with the family dog.

But rabbits as pets have some drawbacks, as well. Their life spans are so much shorter than a dog's or a cat's, averaging five or six years, that loving families experience the awful sting of loss much more quickly. They also hide their illnesses to a much greater degree than do dogs or cats. Since in the wild — and domestic rabbits are closer to the wild than most companion animals — a sick bunny is quickly picked off by predators, masking their illnesses is an important survival strategy for rabbits. But it makes treating them all the more difficult. A bunny that acts sick is a sick bunny indeed. In some cases, by the time they are showing symptoms, it is too late to intervene.

Add to this the fact that we don't know as much about rabbit diseases as we do about the diseases of other species and that, since many rabbits are considered of little monetary value, families do not often choose to invest much in their care, and you can see why we vets treat few rabbits. And rabbits are not good patients. They are designed for one thing — hopping. This they do very well, but their spines are so weak and their thigh and back muscles are so strong that they are liable, with one mighty kick, to literally break their own backs. You would think they would know this about themselves and take strict precautions to prevent it. But during the heart-racing stress of a physical examination by strange white-coated people, they have been known to do exactly that — a fact which makes examining them exceedingly tense.

I have known a few rabbit enthusiasts over the years whose devotion to and love for their pets has been legendary, and who have allowed me to practice quite sophisticated rabbit medicine. At the very top of this short list is Sue Anne Montgomery. Sue Anne is an attractive woman in an earthy sort of way. She has long, straight, dark hair that settles around her shoulders and reaches to the middle of her back. She is thin and shapely, with a pleasant, sun-darkened face. She works as a food producer on a small plot of land supplying vegetables and fruit to the local produce market. She keeps a few head of beef cattle and some goats, which supply the milk from which she makes cheese. A couple of horses are also part of her menagerie and add to her long list of daily chores. This is hard work, and though you can see the effort in her strong and seasoned hands, she still somehow maintains an appealing feminine quality.

Sue Anne used another veterinarian to care for the health needs of her farm animals. But she had a passion for rabbits that elevated them well above the agricultural purposes for which she had begun keeping them. They were her pets. They lived in her house and shared her life in ways most often reserved for the family dog. For these family members, she wanted health care from a family doctor. She brought her bunnies to me.

I suppose I saw four or five of her pet bunnies over the years, but there was one rabbit that was Sue Anne's absolute favorite. Meisha was a female Angora with long hair and a personality that set her apart. I saw her often, as she needed to have her incisor teeth clipped periodically. Rabbits have continuously growing teeth, which, if they do not meet precisely, will overgrow, making it impossible to chew or eat. A quick snip with a sharp clipper keeps them from causing problems, so Meisha came in every four to six weeks.

On one such trip, Sue Anne asked me to check out a little lump she had noticed on

Meisha's tummy. It was the size of a pea and nonpainful, but it had been getting larger over the two-week period she had been watching it. This history alarmed me. Rabbits have a relatively high rate of tumors, and I was concerned that this was a malignancy of the mammary tissue.

"Sue Anne," I said, "I think you should leave Meisha with me today and let me remove that growth."

"Oh, I think that's probably an overreaction, don't you? It's just a little thing. Why don't I just keep an eye on it?"

"We can, if that's what you want, but I would recommend it be removed."

"Do you think it's something serious?" Sue Anne's eyes rounded and concern rose on her face.

"I think it could be. I won't know for sure without a biopsy, but I'm concerned about breast cancer."

The words could not have had more of an impact on Sue Anne had I told her the bank was foreclosing on her mortgage. Immediately, her face clouded over and the precipitation began. She scooped Meisha up in her arms and buried her face in the long silky hair. They stayed that way for what seemed a long time before Sue Anne turned to me again, resolve now marking her face.

"Okay, get that thing off of there right away! I'm glad I brought her in."

Anesthesia in rabbits is a tricky thing and is not to be trifled with. The species is so tenuous that the specter of putting one under the knife is something that gives me nightmares. But I knew that if I was right, Meisha's best chance was for me to remove the growth as soon as possible. That afternoon I took her to surgery and removed the small nodule, making sure to remove a wide swath of normal tissue surrounding it so no tumor cells remained. I also spayed her, in the hope that removal of the ovarian hormones would decrease the likelihood of recurrence. Fortunately, Meisha came through surgery well and was released into the capable and loving care of Sue Anne that evening.

When the biopsy came back from the lab five days later, I was disappointed, although not surprised, to see that the growth had indeed been a malignant tumor of mammary origin. The tissue surrounding the growth had been free of cancer cells, so I hoped that removal had been curative. Time would tell. News of the results produced in Sue Anne the same terrified but resolved response. I gave her instructions to watch the area carefully for any sign of regrowth.

Three months later, Sue Anne and Meisha were back. The record said I was to check another growth. Sue Anne's face showed the fear in her heart as soon as I entered the room.

"Another nodule?" I asked.

Sue Anne just nodded her head, avoiding my face with her frightened and emotion-filled eyes. I took Meisha from her lap and placed her on mine, cupping my hand under her belly and feeling along the mammary chain where the first growth had been. I could feel the surgery scar but did not feel a lump under it. When I went to the other side, however, my heart jumped. There, along a line of mammary tissue on the opposite side, I felt not one nodule but three.

"Oh, Meisha," I said. "That's not good."

Any control Sue Anne had maintained until then evaporated in a torrent of emotion, which continued unabated for quite some time. I sat silently on my stool, patting her arm empathetically. I knew the immensity of the impact this was having on her. No words I could share would lessen it. Finally, Sue Anne turned a tear-streaked face to me and entreated in a pinched voice. "What do we do now?" she asked.

"There really isn't much at our disposal," I said sadly. "These tumors are not very responsive to chemotherapy in other species, and a rabbit does not handle chemo drugs well anyway. Removing the tumors would not help. Since these came back in a different location, I suspect others would just pop up somewhere else. Besides, she can't undergo a whole lot more surgery. I think we only have one option. We'll just keep her as comfortable as possible till the tumors get so large that we can't control her pain. Then we'll have to make an awful decision for her good."

I sent Sue Anne home with pain medications and my deepest sympathies. I wasn't sure how much time she still had with her friend, but I knew it would not be long. Unfortunately, my suspicions turned out to be correct. Within about a month, Sue Anne and Meisha were back for their final visit.

The room was somber when I walked into it that fateful day. Sue Anne sat on the corner bench in a pair of blue jeans, her legs curled up under her. Her head was down and her long hair fell like a curtain over her lap, where Meisha lay, her breath coming now in short gasps. Sue Anne didn't speak when I entered the room, but her shoulders began to shake. Taking my cues from her, I sat down on the stool, scooted it close, and put a hand on her shoulder. After an extended silence broken only by Sue Anne's sniffling and Meisha's labored breathing, I spoke.

"It's time, huh?"

Sue Anne just nodded her head, the tears continuing. She let her legs swing to the floor and handed Meisha to me. I took her and placed her on the exam table. Sue Anne rose and stood on the other side of the table, comforting the frightened bunny with quiet words and gentle touches. The difference from when I had last seen Meisha was remarkable. The tumors, which had been the size of peas then, now ranged in size from golf balls to baseballs, stretching the skin over them and making it difficult for Meisha to move. From her labored breathing, I knew that the tumors had either invaded her lungs or were now causing so much pain that she continuously grunted with discomfort. Either scenario was untenable. As Sue Anne knew, it was definitely time to ease the suffering Meisha was experiencing.

I drew the euthanasia solution into a syringe, anxiety flooding my mind. Rabbits have the tiniest of veins, a fact that makes it very difficult to administer intravenous medications. I did not want this procedure to be prolonged by futile efforts at hitting a vein. With Meisha now back in Sue Anne's embrace, I shaved her ear so I could easily see the minuscule veins that ran along the periphery of the huge ear. They were no bigger than a thread as they snaked their blue way under the skin. It would be difficult to hit this vein in the best of circumstances, but with the swirling emotions of the day, I knew this task to be well nigh impossible.

With Meisha cuddled on the tabletop in Sue Anne's trembling arms, I poised my needle over the vein. Carefully penetrating the thin skin with the needle, I held my breath as I advanced it into the tiny vessel. I was pleasantly surprised to see the solution flow from my syringe into the vein as I slowly pushed the plunger. I had hit the vein. As the fluid flowed into Meisha's system, her breathing slowed and her little body relaxed in Sue Anne's arms. It was a peaceful and dignified end to many years of devotion. I slipped the needle from the vein and placed my stethoscope over the rabbit's slowing heart. Before long, I heard the steady rhythm stop. She was gone.

Sue Anne searched my face as I listened, her breath held in like the emotion I knew was roiling inside. I met her eyes and nodded solemnly. There was silence for a moment. Then from across the table there arose a slow and growing moan of anguish from a crushed heart. Her knees began to buckle and she began to sag down, as if she were bearing more weight than her strength would allow. Her eyes shifted up in their sockets, as if she was searching the ceiling for a rational response to the unanswerable question of why we must endure such loss. Meisha began to slip from her loosening grip.

It was at this point that things began to take a totally unexpected swing into the surreal. I raced around the table and took the deceased rabbit from her arms. Sue Anne's consciousness was rapidly deserting her, and I knew that in just a moment or two, she would be an inert form on the floor if I didn't help.

I directed her with my free hand back to the corner bench and helped her sink down onto it, all the time repeating her name loudly and as comfortingly as I could. I watched with horror as the color drained from her face and her lips formed voiceless words of sadness. The tears fell unchecked from her unseeing eyes.

I knelt on the floor in front of her with the bunny's limp form cradled in the crook of my left arm. I bent over so I could look directly into Sue Anne's face. Since she was huddled forward, I had to lower myself well below the level of her shoulders to look up at her. I could not get her to open her eyes and acknowledge me, even though I was patting her hand with some force. In her unresponsive state, I could not tell whether she was simply overcome with emotion or truly slipping from consciousness.

"Sue Anne," I said, and then, louder, "Sue Anne. Can you hear me?"

Apparently, she could not, because about that time, she slumped forward, unresponsive now. Because I was still holding Meisha's body in my left hand, I had no way to slow her fall except to catch her head on my shoulder and reflexively push her back against the wall with my torso, an action that resulted in my body's being suddenly and uncomfortably close to hers. With my right hand, I reached around and began to rub her back comfortingly yet firmly, hoping with this contact to bring her back to a level of awareness.

As I vigorously rubbed her back, it struck me like a lightning bolt that I did not feel any bra straps. Sue Anne was not wearing a bra! Sue Anne was not wearing a bra? The compromising situation I found myself in suddenly hit me with a clarity that made me back away from the inert body, which was even now cradled on my shoulder in an intimate embrace. I jerked my hand up and back behind me. When I did, though, she slumped again toward the floor, and I had no choice but to move in toward her again. It was either that or let her sink, helpless, to the floor.

I nearly panicked. I envisioned the headlines that would be seen when the news hit the community. VETERINARIAN ABUSES AN UNCONSCIOUS CLIENT AFTER KILLING HER BUNNY. I would be a pariah, a felon. I would no doubt lose my license, my practice, maybe even my family. My clients would desert me in droves. My staff would revolt. My career would be over. *What to do?*

It was about lunchtime on a Wednesday and the office was nearly empty. With no other clients in the building, my receptionist was downstairs in the break room eating her lunch and waiting for me to complete my awful task. I felt very alone. Still not able to rouse Sue Anne from her stupor, I mustered my strength and began to call the receptionist.

"Beth," I called. When there was no answer, my calls grew progressively louder and more frantic. Before long I was bellowing at full voice through the closed door,

Sue Anne, still unperturbed and unhearing, nestled on my shoulder like a mistress. "BETH . . . BETH!"

Finally the door of the exam room opened and Beth entered. I don't know what exactly she expected to find when she opened the door, but from the look on her astonished face, I was sure this loving embrace was not it. Embarrassed, she started to close the door again, apparently to afford us a measure of privacy. I watched the look on her face change from shock to confusion, which transfixed her for a moment before she spoke.

"Which one of you called me?"

This question struck me as incredibly unnecessary under the circumstances. Of the three individuals in the room, I was the only one capable of speech. One was clearly unconscious on my shoulder, and the other was dead in my arm.

"Who do you think called you, Beth?" I snapped.

She stood at the door, unsure whether to enter the room, indecision cloaking her face.

"Did you need something?"

"Yes, Beth, I need your help. Doesn't it appear like I need a little help at this moment?"

Still she stood there as if glued to the

floor, making no movement to come to my aid.

"What do you want me to do?" she asked tentatively.

"Why don't you start by taking the rabbit from my left arm and putting it on the table. Then come and take Sue Anne off my shoulder."

When the reality of what was happening came clear to her, she began to move more quickly. In no time she had Sue Anne laid out on the floor and was bathing her face with cool water and a clean towel. Even so, smelling salts wafted under her nose were required to bring her fully around.

I tried to stay clear of Sue Anne during the forty-five minutes or so it took for her to recover adequately enough to drive her pickup home. I did sneak in a time or two to express again my deepest sympathies at her loss and try to furtively discern whether or not she had any memories of the period during which she was unconscious or if she harbored any intentions to pursue legal action against me. But she was only grateful for my sympathy and saddened by her loss.

It was not until she had gone and the intensity of the emotions had waned that the humor of the situation began to sink in. Every time I pictured myself in that room with one dead rabbit and one pretty girl in a dead faint, both of whom were wrapped in my helpless arms, I broke into laughter.

Wednesday was my afternoon off, and I had arranged to go golfing with three good friends. As we drove to the golf course, I found myself involuntarily smiling to myself again as I reviewed the events of the morning. Just when I was ready to tell the story to my friends, I happened to glance at the pickup truck we were passing. It was pulling a stock trailer and traveling slowly. Absentmindedly, I glanced at the driver — and froze! Instinctively, I sank as deeply as possible into the seat and turned my face away from the truck.

"Don't look at that truck!" I screamed, suddenly frantic.

The car went strangely silent, my friends confused now and looking at me as I hunkered down in the seat. With my hand obscuring my face and my head down, I'm sure I looked like a fugitive at an FBI picnic. My face turned pasty white and my mouth went dry.

"What in the dickens has gotten into you?" one of my friends asked.

"That truck," I yelled in response. "Pass it, quick . . . and don't look at the driver!"

In an incredible twist of fate, we had happened upon this truck, and I had recognized the woman driving! With her long, dark hair, she was very familiar to me. She was driving slowly, her head hanging sadly and her hand clutching a Kleenex, with which she dabbed at her weeping eyes. It was Sue Anne!

WILLIAM

My history is imbued with richness — not monetary wealth so much — but after eighteen-plus years in the same small town, there is much texture and color woven into my memories. I find it odd that my memories of two decades of life diminish the difficult times and wreathe the good ones in garlands of glowing gladness. I still smart at the significant losses, of course, but the day-to-day annoyances and frustrations are mostly gone now as I think back. What remains in my mind are the bright patches of emotional color that make up the quilt of my experience.

Much of this richness accrues by virtue of the personalities and characters of the people whose pets I have treated over the years and whose experiences and memories intertwine with mine. At any one time, there is a matrix of such people whose dogs and cats make up my patient list. But because some patients pass on and because people change jobs and locations, the makeup of that matrix is constantly in flux. When a special client slips from the network, it is with nostalgia that I recall that person and the place of prominence he or she once held in my professional world. I was reminded yesterday of one special personality, whose memory always brings a fond smile.

Susan met me in the treatment room one day with a cat carrier, from which she extracted a cat of the Siamese denomination. Though close observation revealed that he might not have actually been Siamese, he did look like a recent convert who was trying hard to become one. His coat was a little longer than that of most Siamese. His coloring was the same, though it lacked the sleek, spoiled sheen typical of the breed. Instead, it had the coarse, rough texture of a cat that made his own way in the world. Neither did he display the confused, cross-eyed Siamese expression; instead, he fixed on me focused eyes of penetrating intelligence. There was about him a certain presence that made me take notice.

"What do you have there, Susan?" I asked with interest.

"An old lady just dropped him off for us to look at. She says he's limping on one of

273

his back legs. She doesn't know exactly what happened, but he came back in after being gone for a few days and was holding up his leg. She says to do whatever is necessary to fix him. She couldn't stay for an examination; said she had some errands to run and to just call her when you have more information."

It was a story pocked with red flags, having all the hallmarks of a dumped cat. I have had cats abandoned at the practice many times over the years by irresponsible people who cared little for the animals that adored them. They typically were too "busy" to wait for me to examine the pet, and left phony names, addresses, and phone numbers. Once the hapless patient was successfully deposited within the confines of the office, the owner would skip and we would never hear from him or her again. With bad information, our attempts at contacting the person would be fruitless. It was how Rush had ended up in my home. What to do with this cat?

"Have we ever seen any of this lady's pets before?"

"No, this is the first one."

"Does this cat have a name?" I asked. Many times, dumped cats come without names or with names in which no creative energy has been invested.

"The lady said his name was William."

"William, huh? Not Bill? That's a big name for a cat. Let's take a look."

I had already been watching William make his way around the room, holding his right hind leg off the ground carefully. I had already noted how it formed an odd angle below the hip and how the foot hung a little too loosely. I already knew William had a broken leg. It was a simple thing to confirm a fracture of the femur with just a quick feel of the bone. There was grating of the broken ends of bone against each other and severe bruising on the inside of the leg. It always amazes me how stoic my patients can be when they sustain injuries that would leave us humans screaming for morphine. William reacted to my probing simply by turning his head and flinching slightly.

The rest of William's examination was unremarkable, if you call the ability to stave off shock and unremitting pain in the face of serious injury unremarkable. In all other respects, William seemed normal. I estimated him to be about three or four years old. He had been neutered, was in good flesh, and free of fleas. He seemed to have been provided with good care. Still, though William seemed okay, reservations about his owner remained.

I fully expected to dial a nonworking number as I lifted the phone to my ear to call the owner. To my surprise, the phone was answered promptly by a woman with a voice that belied many years of experience and also an impressive degree of education and sophistication. Hers was a deep voice, not only in tone but in character. My concerns were allayed.

"Is this Mrs. Moynihan?"

"It certainly is. Who is this?"

"I'm Dr. Coston, ma'am. You just left your kitty, William, at our hospital."

"Oh, yes. Thank you for calling so quickly. William is such a dear. What's wrong with poor William?"

"He has a broken leg."

"I was afraid of that. You know, he's such an independent soul. He absolutely insists upon going outside and roaming the neighborhood while we're out here in the Fort. He stays inside when we're in the city. But here, he just must be let outside. I was afraid he'd get hurt at some point. And now he's gone and done it. What do we need to do to get William back on his feet again, so to speak?" She laughed easily at her play on words.

I knew without explanation that "the city"

was Washington, D.C. There was an ease of interaction, an assumption of acceptance about her that I sensed had arisen from living among the privileged who resided in the stately 1930s- and 1940s-era homes within the Beltway, not from the straining ambition teeming in the northern Virginia suburbs. No doubt she was one of the many D.C. residents who sought serenity on the weekends and in their retirement years in the quietude of the outer reaches of Shenandoah County.

I learned later that Mrs. Moynihan and her husband had purchased St. David's Church, a crumbling piece of history in the Fort that was slowly bowing to the ravages of time, and had restored it bit by bit to a place of rustic beauty that served as their getaway. Not only had the church been converted by their loving attentions but each of the outbuildings had undergone physical and spiritual transformations as well, till the site was once again a scene of tranquil elegance. You can still see the Moynihans' craftsmanship if you drive east on St. David's Church Road in Fort Valley. It will be on the left. You'll recognize it.

"I haven't taken X-rays yet, so I don't know for sure what he'll need. But I'm almost certain he'll need surgery to repair the bone. Breaks in this location almost always do."

"Well, I have complete confidence in your judgment. You do whatever William needs to get him well again. Just let me know when to pick him up. We miss him here at the homestead."

It struck me that she was expressing such confidence in me even though we had never met and this phone conversation was the first we'd ever had. Rather than making me uncomfortable, though, it filled me with determination to warrant the confidence she was placing in me.

"I suppose we should talk about the expense of the surgery, Mrs. Moynihan."

"You can if you'd like, Doctor. I know a surgery like that is pretty involved. But my William is worth whatever it is you must charge me to fix him. I'm not worried about that even a little bit. I hope you won't worry about it, either."

And on nothing more than her word, I did not. It is a rare gift indeed for a veterinarian to receive — a client who places such high value on her relationship with her four-legged family members and is blessed with the financial wherewithal to provide, without concern for the costs, the medical care her pets need. Not every person who shares with Mrs. Moynihan her love for a pet can do so. And not all who can afford the care share Mrs. Moynihan's unqualified devotion to a pet. In the many years between when I first met William and when the Moynihans moved back to the city, I have treated a host of her cats. Never has it been necessary to factor costs into the calculus of their medical care.

That afternoon I took William to surgery. The X-rays showed a fracture in the middle of the femur, with a spiral curve to the bone ends that would allow placement of stainless-steel pins and wires to stabilize it. The X-rays made it look like a routine repair. They often do. But once the incision was made, things looked different, what with the bruising and tissue damage.

From the fracture site, I inserted pins into the middle of the bone, driving them toward the hip and exiting them out of the bone at the top of the leg. Attaching a driving device, I then pulled them up farther into the bone's center, till their tips were even with the broken edges of the bone. Then, after fitting the fracture pieces together like a glistening white puzzle, I drove the pins down into the center of the bone in the lower half of the femur, below the fracture, seating them firmly in the dense bone just

279

above the knee. This prevented the abnormal bending at the fracture site, but it did nothing to prevent the bone ends from rotating around the pins. Placing three wires a centimeter or two apart and twisting them tightly around the bone fragments did. What remained was to cut off the remainder of the pins, which extended above the hip, and to close the tissues with sutures. In an hour and a half, the surgery was done. Postoperative X-rays showed a good repair of the fracture, the pins and wires standing out on the film in stark relief to the surrounding bone and soft tissue. The fact that the top of the pins extended farther above the bone in the hip than I would have liked gave me a moment's pause, but overall I was pleased with my handiwork.

We set William up in a cage, the fluids dripping into his arm flooding him with waves of pain medications and sedatives while he slowly regained his senses. I left the office with a feeling of accomplishment that evening. I had been a good veterinarian.

I have found it interesting over the years that even though most days end like this, they are offset by a few days when the overarching feeling is a sense of failure, a nagging suspicion that somehow I've breached my contract with my patients, that I've been more of a menace to them than their advocate. I suppose every professional is burdened with sporadic feelings of inadequacy. But since my patients are so dependent and utterly voiceless, those days for me are especially brutal. So it was an especially good thing to turn the lights off and leave the office with a successful surgery under my belt and a recovering patient in his cage.

I was not expecting what I found the next morning. William greeted me with a mournful yowl and nonstop hissing when I opened his cage door. I had not known him long, but I was quite sure this was not his normal demeanor. When I placed him carefully on the ground, I was pleased to see that he was walking on his operated leg, but with each step he screamed in pain and turned with confusion to bite at his hip.

I suspected that the tips of the pins which extended above the bone on his hip were too long. With each step, the three-quarters of an inch of stainless steel impinged upon the sciatic nerve, trapping it against the pelvis and causing intense sciatica. It took only a few minutes with William anesthetized again to snip off another half inch or more of each pin and, using a surgical hammer, to tap the pin ends gently, seating them again deeper into the bone. In an hour, William was fully awake and walking around the room with barely a limp, an organized row of neatly spaced sutures decorating the side of his leg.

Mrs. Moynihan came to pick William up later that afternoon. My first impression of her had already been formed during our phone conversation. Meeting her only confirmed those perceptions. She was tall and willowy, with silver hair, dark-rimmed glasses, and a smile that was open and engaging. She was dressed in a long cotton flower-print skirt and a blouse of pastel green. A simple string of pearls and matching pearl bracelets and earrings completed the ensemble. She was thrilled that William had been restored to health and was enthralled by the before and after X-rays that I showed her.

William went on to recover from his injury, and just a few weeks later, he was back for a recheck appointment. X-rays showed that the fracture had healed completely; the bone at the fracture site was even stronger now than it had been originally. Even his hair had grown in fully. During a quick anesthetic procedure, I removed the pins that had allowed the bones to heal so perfectly, leaving the three wires encircling the now-whole bone.

After William, Mrs. Moynihan entrusted the care of CeeCee and several other cats to me. In the nine or ten years I treated her animals, I found Mrs. Moynihan always to be the same — perfectly dressed, pleasant, sophisticated, arty, always ready with a laugh and a compliment, and armed each time I saw her with a new joke to share, most of them innocently off-color, an ironic twist to the otherwise-refined woman that she was.

And then suddenly, Mrs. Moynihan came to the office no more. Through other clients, I learned that her husband had aged to the point that closer proximity to their health-care providers was prudent. They had put the old church up for sale and some lucky family had purchased a visionary couple's dream, resplendent with finery and character. On a trip back to the area many months later, Mrs. Moynihan stopped by the office. She was driving a brand-new pastel blue Volkswagen Bug with a fresh carnation sitting in a small vase on the dashboard. In her typical easy manner and her husky, musical voice, she told me that William had passed away at the respectable age of seventeen, still, like her, in possession of his singular pride and carriage. She brought with her an Art Deco print of a willowy Parisian girl portrayed with a wispy, long-haired Saluki by her side. I cherish that picture and the wonderful memories it evokes. It still hangs prominently in my office. I think of Mrs. Moynihan each time I see it and smile.

So here's to you, Mrs. Moynihan, and to William and CeeCee. Here's to all the clients and patients that have made their way into and out of the halls of my office and my memory. I live my life in gratitude for the remarkable privilege my clients have bestowed upon me in entrusting the care of their pets to me, of including me as an integral thread in the intricate weave of their relationship with them, of joining the emotional ebb and flow of their lives with mine for a time. Cheers to you all!

Playing Keno

I can remember few patients in the course of my professional life that looked as sick as Keno did when I walked into the examination room one morning. A four-year-old female rottweiler, Keno was usually an imposing presence, despite her pussy cat personality. The square, muscular head and jowls, the penetrating intensity of her gaze, and the reputation of her breed made me proceed cautiously the first time we met. However, as is true of most of my rotty patients, who are so often assumed to be guilty of man-eating tendencies, Keno possessed not a single mean gene. She preferred to slather you with slobbery kisses, her front feet planted solidly on your shoulders, rather than intimidate you with her considerable size. Still, at ninety-five pounds, her presence filled the exam room completely. Not so that morning, however.

I found her lying flat on her side, ignoring

my entrance. She did not even lift her head or raise her ears. It seemed all she could do just to follow my movements with her sad eyes, the nub of her tail still. On the bench in the corner sat Steph Malnotti, her face white with concern. Steph and her husband, Tim, were regular clients who owned three massive rottweilers. Since they were childless, these three dogs held places of high honor in the Malnotti household. I knew from our discussions that attempts at adding a child to the family had met with disappointment and had elevated the dogs to almost offspring status. As I stood looking at Keno, my mind already contemplating the possible diagnoses, Steph's face clouded with emotion and she started to cry.

"Oh Dr. C.," she said between quaking sobs, "she's really bad. I should have brought her in a couple days ago. She didn't seem that bad until last night. But by then your office was closed. Is she too far gone?"

"I don't know yet, Steph," I said, trying to present an optimistic front despite the gathering gloom I was feeling. "When did Keno start to feel bad?"

"She hasn't eaten much in the last five or six days. I thought it was the new food I had changed her to, so I didn't worry much about it. But three days ago she started vomiting and her appetite dropped to nothing. Yesterday, though, she got worse, and this morning she was really bad."

I knelt on the floor and lifted Keno's lips. Her gums were sticky and dry and a bright brick red color. I gently bunched an inch or two of skin over her shoulder between my fingers, pulled it away from the underlying tissues, and released it. It took three or four seconds for it to fall back to its normal position, another indication of dehydration. I listened to her rapid heartbeat through my stethoscope, timing it with my watch to a rate of 160 beats a minute. Keno was in shock. With the bell of my stethoscope over her lung fields, I listened to the rapid inflow and outflow of air. The respirations were way too fast, as well.

I slipped a digital thermometer into her rectum and watched the numbers on the display begin to rise rapidly, spinning ever upward like an electronic gambling machine. While I waited, I pieced together the information I had gleaned so far: rapid respiration, brick red gum color, dehydration, profound lethargy. . . . Just then, the high-pitched beep of the digital thermometer went off and I looked at the display. I added a temperature of 105.4 degrees to the list of signs. It looked like Keno had septic shock, a condition brought on by systemic infection. But where was the source?

Throughout my initial assessment, Keno remained lying down, barely responding to the things I had done. But when I slid my left hand underneath her belly and pressed down toward it with my right hand on top, she reacted with a yelp of pain, turning her head to me with indignation. That effort was all she could make, and her head dropped again, her cheek hitting the floor with a loud *thunk*. I repeated the maneuver to see if her tummy really hurt that much or if she had simply wearied of my probing. Her reaction was the same. She was clearly in pain when I applied any degree of pressure to her abdomen. As I released my hands, I noticed a little ripple rebound along her stomach, like waves on a puddle when you step in it. This fluid wave was not a good omen. Despite her obvious discomfort, I needed to examine her abdomen more thoroughly.

"Hey, Steph, hold her head down on the floor while I feel her belly better, please." Steph bent to her task, one that was made that much easier by the appalling weakness of the patient.

Carefully, I palpated Keno's abdomen,

starting just in front of her rear legs and working my way forward. Her discomfort was most pronounced as I reached the front end of her belly and gently probed under her rib cage. I leaned back on my heels and faced Steph as she released Keno's head and slumped back onto the bench, her body language reflecting my concern.

"Steph," I said, choosing my words carefully, "Keno has what we call an acute abdomen. That is not a diagnosis so much as it is a description. An acute abdomen simply means that there is significant pain and discomfort in the abdomen. It can be caused by any number of things, from blunt trauma to pancreatitis to tumor to foreign-body ingestion. But acute abdomen generally means we need to go in surgically and find out what is going on."

"Okay," Steph said without hesitation, "let's do whatever we have to do to save her."

"I'm glad you're good with that," I replied hesitantly, "but there are some strikes against us here that may make this more complicated. She has a very high fever, it appears that she's got fluid in her belly, and she's in shock. Those things in addition to the acute abdomen make me concerned about sepsis." I could tell from Steph's blank look that this made no sense to her.

"What is sepsis?"

"It means that she also has active infection throughout her system. With the fluid in the belly, I'm concerned that the cause of her sepsis is peritonitis — an infection in her abdominal cavity. If that's the case, then there could be a rupture of the bowel somewhere, and that is a very serious condition. I won't know till I get in there, but if there is peritonitis, the likelihood of Keno's recovering may be pretty low. If we were just playing the odds, I wouldn't bet any money on it."

Steph was quiet for a moment as she considered the sobering words. Then she turned to me hopefully. "Is there no chance at all?"

"Well, again, I won't know for sure until I get into surgery. But if it is really peritonitis, the chances are low."

"Are they zero?"

"I wouldn't say zero, but probably less than twenty percent."

Steph fidgeted in her seat, her eyes searching the floor around where Keno still lay motionless. "I'll have to talk to Tim for sure, but I know what he'll say. Keno was named for a game of chance. And I know we will want to give her that chance if there's any hope at all. You get started and I'll call Tim and talk it through with him. If he thinks we should quit, I'll call you."

"I don't know what part finances play in your thinking, Steph. But this could be expensive."

"Yeah, I figured as much. Tim and I will discuss that, too. But unless you hear from us, plan on doing whatever is necessary."

Because Keno was too weak to walk on her own, I got a stretcher and, with Lisa's help, carried her back into my treatment room. I drew some blood for testing, got some X-rays, and started intravenous fluids to combat the dehydration and shock. I blasted her with powerful antibiotics and gave medications for pain. The X-rays confirmed fluid accumulation in Keno's abdomen, and the blood work showed a dramatic elevation in the white-cell count. Keno's system was mustering all available soldiers to fight off the invading bacteria.

Within an hour or so, I had Keno in the surgery room and was incising through her skin, the surgery lights blazing over my shoulder. As I lifted the abdominal wall with forceps and cut through the body wall, I was met with a gush of foul-smelling reddish fluid that erupted from the wound and spilled across my sterile drapes and onto the floor. My heart sank — peritonitis! The flow of the sickly reddish yellow fluid continued unabated. I had to empty perhaps two or three gallons of the stuff before I could even begin to assess the abdominal cavity. When I finally achieved a clear field, it was obvious that the internal organs were suffering ill effects. Instead of having the glistening pink surface of normal intestines, Keno's intestines were red and enflamed and injected with tiny vessels that throbbed and oozed.

With my gloved fingers, I felt along the entire course of the intestines, starting at the south end and working my way upstream. Not finding any foreign material present, I turned my attention to the stomach. I first located the spot at which the esophagus enters the stomach on the left side. Then I felt along the bulging curves of the stomach, where the bulk of a meal is stored. I could identify nothing other than the residue of the last meal Keno had eaten, almost a week ago, which still had not passed out of the distended organ.

As I followed the stomach to its outflow tract with my fingers, I bumped against something firm. Sure enough, down deep, where the pylorus dived almost out of reach below the right lobe of the liver, I could feel something hard and rubbery. In fact, as I curled my hand around the region, I could make out several similar pieces of the same substance wedged into much too small a space, completely obstructing the passage of food. Something else, too, made my blood run cold. As I grasped the affected tissue gently in my hand and pulled it closer to the surface, I noticed an area of ugly dark purple tissue that looked mostly devitalized over where the foreign material was firmly wedged in place.

Even more disconcerting was the slimy yellowish fluid that oozed through a rent in the middle of this angry, bruised intestinal wall. This was the source of the infection in the abdominal cavity. And it was my worst nightmare. Not only had the intestine ruptured, but it had done so in perhaps the worst-possible location. That region of the duodenum, which was the most inaccessible and also the place where the pancreatic and bile ducts emptied, would have to be removed and reconstructive techniques employed to restore as normal a digestive function as possible. It would be a dicey bit of surgery, fraught with a host of possible complications and a high risk of catastrophic failure. It was a race I was destined to lose — one in which I was handicapped beyond description by the inescapable fact that Keno's raging peritonitis had already beaten me to the punch.

Before proceeding with drastic surgery, I had Lisa dial the Malnottis' number and hold the phone to my ear. I described what I had found upon entering the abdomen, the worst-case-scenario foreign body in the duodenum, and the surgical techniques required to give Keno even the slightest hope. I warned of the potential outcome, the difficulty of the recovery period, and the likelihood of significant financial investment in this difficult fight. But despite my tale of gloom, I was instructed to spare no expense in Keno's care.

I proceeded to remove a sizable portion of her duodenum, fishing out of the damaged section of intestine several pieces of the tennis ball that had occluded Keno's intestines for almost a week. I then sewed the remaining intestinal wall closed, trying my best to salvage the ductwork that drained the gallbladder and pancreas. Then I flushed the abdomen liberally with eight or ten liters of warmed saline solution, until the fluid I removed after each liter ran clear.

Finally, with my shirt soaked with sweat and my back hunched in what felt like a permanent Notre Dame–worthy stance, I placed the final suture in the skin and pushed back from the surgery table. The procedure had taken close to three hours and I was physically and emotionally drained. There is a saying among surgeons: "The solution to pollution is dilution." But despite being guilty of extreme overkill in the dilution category, I was not confident that the pollution problem had been solved. Nor was I sure that the damaged intestinal wall I had sutured was healthy enough to heal. Time would tell. I was still not betting on Keno.

For the next several days I flooded Keno's system with many liters of intravenous fluids, thousands of milligrams of powerful antibiotics, and enough pain medications to render her an addict. Her attitude improved daily, though her appetite did not return. By the weekend she was better, although still in need of intensive therapy, so I referred her to the twenty-four-hour veterinary-care facility thirty minutes away. All weekend I could think of little else, rehashing each step of the surgery and her aftercare. Had there been anything else I could have done to help her get better?

On Monday morning Tim Malnotti brought Keno back to my hospital. I went out to his car to help him carry her into the hospital. The moment I saw her, though, I knew her condition had deteriorated.

"Oh, Tim, she doesn't look good at all! I can just see it in her eyes."

"Yeah, that's what I thought when I saw her this morning, too. What should we do?"

"She needs more intensive care than I can provide in my hospital. She may, in fact, need more surgery. And if that's the case, then I think it should be done by specialists. If you still want to proceed, I think we should refer her to the veterinary school in Blacksburg."

"Okay, you make the call. I'm going to get on the road."

"Tim," I said, "you should know that this might be expensive."

"I appreciate your concern, but now's not the time to stop."

While I made a call to the veterinary school, Tim headed down the road for the three-hour trip to Blacksburg, where the Virginia-Maryland Regional College of Veterinary Medicine was situated on one corner of the Virginia Tech campus. During the ten days she was hospitalized, the doctors there had to go back in and remove even more of her duodenum, reroute the outflow tract of her stomach, and remove her gallbladder. But after the second surgery, her recovery was steady. Though for the rest of her life Keno required supplementation of pancreatic enzymes and vitamins, she was otherwise healthy.

You would think after the mess she had placed herself in, Keno would have learned not to consume recreational equipment. But four or five weeks after she had recovered from this episode, she was back in my hospital, showing similar symptoms. I was forced to do a third surgery, during which I again removed the hemispheres of another tennis ball she had eaten. Since we were able to intervene much earlier the second time, the surgery and Keno's recovery from it was much less dramatic.

At the time of suture removal from the final surgery, I turned to Tim and Steph. "You guys should be commended for all the care you have given Keno. She really struck the jackpot when you adopted her. Not many families would have been able to give her all the care you have. I know this whole episode has cost you a fortune."

"You're right, Doc C.," Tim replied. "I added up all the bills from this the other night and it totaled a little more than ten thousand dollars."

"Wow, that's a lot! Well, I'm glad she's finally back to normal now. I wouldn't have bet a nickel on her when I saw her that first morning. Was it worth all that money?"

"We have no regrets at all," Tim said. Steph nodded her head in agreement. "In fact, I've been meaning to ask you. When you called us during surgery that first day to say that it looked bad and gave us the option of putting her down, were you serious?"

"Absolutely. In my business, many, if not most, of my clients would have done just that, given the seriousness of her disease and the costs of treating her. Those choosing to proceed would have made the choice on the next Monday morning or before the surgery down at Tech. You guys are the exception to the rule."

The Malnottis were quiet for few moments, considering my words. Then Tim turned to me again. "That amazes us, Doc C. Our dogs are our children. We would no more have considered putting Keno to sleep when there was any chance at all for her to recover than we would have euthanized our baby. We are fortunate that we can afford her care. But we still would have done this if we had been forced to mortgage our home."

"Keno is one lucky dog!"

The Malnottis are still good friends of

mine, though Keno and her cohorts are now gone, victims of old age. Tim and Steph are now too busy to have dogs in their home. Three pregnancies later, they are now the proud parents of four children, who occupy every spare second. But I cannot forget the roll of the dice that they took with Keno, for on the wall of my office hangs a plaque that Tim and Steph presented to me after Keno was fully recovered. On it is a picture of Keno with a sloppy grin and bright eyes. In her mouth is clamped a tennis ball, very possibly one of the two tennis balls I removed from her over the course of those two long months. Below her picture are these words:

> You are my hero and trusted friend
> You have been blessed with the ability to
>   mend
> I swallowed my ball and you took it out
> You saved my life without a doubt
> I came to you broken and sick
> And I thanked you with a wag and a lick

MY GIRLFRIEND MEGAN

"Dr. Coston, I think my dog has broken her leg."

The voice was even and measured, but I could sense the concern lurking just below the surface. Ms. Elaine Farmer had been a client for a year or two, and I knew her and her dogs well. Elaine was educated, level-headed, and unswervingly devoted to her dogs, Megan and Max. Though she was controlling the fear and panic well, I could tell she was distraught.

"Tell me what happened, Elaine." Often an owner's first assessment of the severity of a problem is exaggerated by her own anxiety, so I usually expect the problem to be less serious than is perceived. I was not concerned yet, especially because Elaine's voice was so calm and controlled.

"Well, the dogs and I were going down to the mailbox this evening. My driveway is almost a mile long, so it's a great walk for all of us. All of a sudden, a pickup came barreling around the corner and ran right over Megan. Now she won't put any weight on the leg, and I think I can see the bone. Will you check her out?"

"Of course I will. Bring her right down. I'll meet you at the office." I was still not terribly alarmed. It's not unusual for a client to see subcutaneous tissues in a wound and assume she is seeing bone. Tendons, ligaments, and muscle sheaths can easily be mistaken for bones by the uninitiated. I felt sure that I would find a less serious injury than Ms. Farmer had described.

At that time in my practice, there was not an emergency hospital available, which meant that I saw my patients on an emergency basis when the situation called for it. Since I didn't have as far to go as Ms. Farmer, I arrived at the hospital before she and Megan did. With my mind running over the possible wounds I might encounter, I turned on the X-ray machine, retrieved bandage materials, and prepared the drugs I thought I might need.

Within a short time, Ms. Farmer rumbled into the parking lot, the motor of her Ford F-150 pickup truck grumbling quietly, like that of an idling motorboat. She lived in the Fort. Her job as a clinical psychologist required her to leave home in even the most inclement of weather — thus the impressive pickup truck with high clearance, four-wheel drive, and an extra-powerful engine. Chrome running boards helped Elaine scale the heights into the driver's seat, as her stature was neither tall nor particularly petite. I recognized the vehicle immediately.

I ran out to the truck, threw open the door, and jumped up onto the running board on the passenger side. Megan was sitting on the front seat, her leg wrapped in a towel. Her face was the picture of pain and anxiety, but she greeted me warmly with a wag of her tail and a broad swipe of her tongue on my cheek.

Megan was a lean sixty-pound Labrador-shepherd cross with a long, fringed tail and flopping ears. Her coat was fairly long, brown and highlighted with wisps of lighter hair ringing her face and eyes, raccoonlike. A splotch of white splattered her chest. Megan had always struck me as a docile and totally agreeable dog, but tonight I was cautious because of her injuries. Gingerly, I lifted her in my arms and stepped as lightly as possible from the running board to the ground. Despite my caution, the step was high and the effect was jarring on Megan's injured leg. She whimpered quietly but otherwise bore her pain without further complaint. I carried her to an examination room and deposited her onto the table.

Quickly I examined her for other injuries. I looked in her mouth, listened to her heart, felt her abdomen, looked in her ears, and manipulated her other limbs carefully, not wanting to focus in too quickly on the obvious problem and miss clues to other internal injuries. Fortunately, everything else seemed to be fine.

Slowly and as gingerly as possible, I unwrapped the towel from the injured leg. As I worked, Megan monitored my every movement, tenderly licking my hands as if to say, "I'm really glad for your help, Doc. But remember, that leg really hurts and I'd appreciate it if you'd go slowly." I thanked her for her kisses and tried as best I could to reassure her with quiet, soothing dialogue. It was working: She trusted me.

As I pulled away the last of the makeshift bandage, I recoiled at the sight. Just above the right wrist was a large, gaping wound, through which protruded about three inches of glistening white bone. The shattered ends of the radius and the ulna, the two bones in the forearm, were coated with blood and debris from the gravel driveway. Grass, dirt, and small sticks clung to their jagged edges and were scattered throughout the wound. Held by the skin and soft tissue around the fracture, the wrist and foot dangled like a plumb bob on the end of the limb. Since no vessels had been damaged, there was surprisingly little blood. Megan looked up at me gamely, almost apologetically, and licked my hand once again.

I was moved with admiration for this noble and courageous creature and awed by her trust in me. For just a moment, I allowed myself to ponder the privilege and responsibility of meriting such unwavering confidence! My heart went out to the valiant dog and I cradled her head in my hands. Bending over, I laid my cheek on her forehead and whispered in her ear.

"Oh, Megan, I'm so sorry you're hurting. We're going to make you feel better, okay? Just work with me and we'll get through this."

Without moving her head, she turned her eyes up to me and, with an amazing clarity of cognizance, gently licked my hands again in an unmistakable reply, never taking her gaze from my eyes. They were just little things really — that lick, those eyes, the expression on her face. But there was in them a universe of meaning. They spoke of pain and confusion. They apologized for inconveniencing me. There was even, perhaps, anger at the careless driver of that pickup. But they mainly told of gratitude and confidence and acceptance, of satisfaction that her care would be in my hands, and of submission to my judgment. And in that moment of connection, I resolved to warrant her confidence. This dog would walk again if it was the last thing I did!

Our reverie lasted only a moment or two before I turned my attention again to the job at hand, almost embarrassed by the display to which Elaine had been privy. I gave Megan a sedative, an antibiotic, medication to fight shock, and a shot for pain. After placing an intravenous catheter and administering fluids and anesthetics, I proceeded to clean the debris off the bone ends. I then manipulated the bones through the wounds and returned them to approximately their normal locations. The fracture was a bad one and would require surgery to align the bones properly and stabilize them with pins and wires. But the middle of the night was not the right time to undertake such an involved procedure. I covered the wound with a temporary bandage, settled Megan into a cage, and continued the flow of intravenous fluids into her system. Then I turned to Ms. Farmer.

"Okay, so tomorrow I'll take her to surgery and see what we can do about fixing that fracture. For tonight, she needs rest and fluids. The pain medications will keep her as comfortable as possible till then. I'll stay with her tonight till she is fully awake."

"So she's gonna be okay?"

"I don't think her life is in danger. That's the good news. But the fracture is a bad one. I don't need X-rays to tell me it's a fracture. But they will tell me how badly mangled the bones are on the other side of the fracture, where I can't see. Once I get those, I'll have a better idea what will be required. Certainly it's going to be a surgical fix. But she's young and a fighter, so I'm hopeful!"

The next day, with the help of my staff, I anesthetized Megan again and took X-rays of her leg. I was pleased to see that the bones beyond the fracture line that joined the wrist were not shattered. Still, with only about an inch or two of bone between the fracture site and the wrist bones, I didn't have much to work with for the surgical repair. During surgery, I fashioned a pair of curving metal pins, which I introduced at the wrists. These entered the hollow center of the bone, crossed the fracture site inside the bone, and bounced off the opposite inner wall, curving and gaining purchase on the inner wall of the side they had entered. With one pin placed on each side, the bones were stabilized and the fracture site was protected. Though the repair had been a difficult one, I was confident the bones would heal.

The surgery had been stressful, and I was tired and wringing with sweat as I placed the last sutures. A metal plate would have been a better fix, no doubt, but I did not have that capability in my hospital, and Elaine had ruled out a referral to a specialist. The repair would have to be augmented with a bandage and splint for a few weeks, but I had kept my promise to Megan.

As she recovered from the effects of the anesthetics, I placed a sturdy plastic splint on the injured leg, then secured it in place with layers of cotton gauze and a stretchable bandage. Covered with a final layer of brightly colored moisture-resistant material over the cotton and sprayed with a mist of bitter-tasting liquid to dissuade her from chewing at it, the bandage was finished. It was bulky and heavy, to be sure. I knew it would take a few days for Megan to become accustomed to it, but I felt certain it would do the job. The rest was up to Megan. She needed rest now and weeks of quiet recuperation.

As I waited for Megan to come around completely from the anesthetics, I called Elaine and explained to her how important it would be for her to curtail Megan's habitually vivacious approach to life. I heard her laugh apologetically into the phone, knowing how difficult a task I had assigned her. Megan was only a year and a half old at the time — still a puppy with a devil-may-care attitude. About that time, Megan, still heavily medicated for pain, lifted her head and wagged her tail. As the clinging fog of the analgesics wore off, I saw relief and the lifting of anxiety in her eyes.

During the next two days, while Megan recovered in the hospital, I noticed a special intensity in her eyes whenever I entered the room. She would attentively follow my motions and perk her ears up at the sound of my voice. Like few other patients in my career, Megan fell for me with a fervency that bordered on fanaticism. It was not just that she liked me. It was more than that. The inescapable fact was that she had a crush on me — like a teenager's infatuation with an attractive teacher. And I was not the only one to notice. Lisa and the rest of the staff were greatly amused and teased me about having a "thing" going on with a patient. I brushed off their humor, flattered by Megan's obvious devotion.

On the third day after surgery, I discharged Megan to Elaine's capable care. I prescribed oral antibiotics and pain medication to ease the postoperative discomfort, and issued stern warnings to keep Megan's activity level strictly curtailed. She was to go outside only on a leash and under careful supervision. Elaine was to keep the bandage dry and clean; this point I stressed at length. Because the bandage was constructed largely of cotton batting under the exterior wrap, any moisture at the toes would wick up the cotton, leaving the inside of the bandage wet. Since the outer layers were moisture-resistant, this wetness would be retained against the skin, increasing the discomfort, causing nasty dermatitis, and dramatically increasing the risk of infection at the surgical site. Then I sent Elaine and Megan home, flush with feelings of accomplishment.

Two days later I got a call from Ms. Farmer. "I'm afraid I've been a bad momma," she said.

"Oh, I doubt that. What happened?"

"Well, Megan got out the back door when I let Max out. And before I noticed she was gone, she was swimming in the creek. The bandage is soaking wet. How do I get it to dry out?"

"You don't," I responded. "If the bandage is that wet, the only option is to bring her in and replace it. If we don't, we'll be sorry, and we'll endanger all that we've accomplished with surgery."

"I was afraid of that. Okay, I'll bring her in."

Megan was thrilled to see me when Elaine brought her in later that day. No reunion between parted lovers was ever more joyful. Her face shone with eagerness and her greeting was effusive as I met her in the lobby. While I removed the sodden mass of dripping cotton from her leg and replaced it with clean and dry bandage material, she lovingly caressed my hand with her paw and licked my arm tenderly. Before I sent them once again on their way, I reiterated my advice to keep her bandage clean and dry.

Despite my instructions to Elaine, and despite her most careful efforts to enforce them, over the next few weeks Megan became an accomplished escape artist. Whenever she was able to sneak out, she headed directly for the creek at the back of the Farmer property and plunged in for a swim, completely saturating the gauze and cotton bandage and necessitating a visit to our office for another bandage change.

Each time, Megan would bound through the front doors, tongue dangling in a sloppy smile and eyes bright with anticipation. When she caught sight of me behind the counter, she would woof excitedly, crouch down playfully, splay-legged, with her wagging hindquarters and flagging tail high in the air. Then she would run full tilt across the lobby, dragging Elaine at the end of the leash, and plop her front legs onto the countertop, complete with a sodden mass of bedraggled bandage.

I would, of course, reward such a shameless display of adoration with the lavish response it deserved. It underscored to me what a lucky breed we veterinarians are. What other doctors can interact with their patients so expressively and not get sued?

The problem was, however, that Megan began to look forward to our reunions altogether too much. In the eleven or twelve weeks after her injury, I replaced that bandage no fewer than ten times. I began to wonder if Megan was purposely soiling her bandage so she could see me again. Bandage changes became so routine for her that I'm sure Megan could have applied the bandage herself. But she wanted me to do it. During each rewrapping of the leg, she would occupy herself with loving, almost amorous, licking of my hands and face, resting her good leg comfortably on my shoulder. With each visit, it was obvious that her puppy love was growing.

After three months, the bones had healed adequately enough for me to remove the pins and wires and leave the bandage off. Megan was walking well, with hardly a trace of a limp, and her visits became infrequent. I missed seeing her so often. The staff teased me about being stood up by my mistress. But I knew better.

Megan was a patient of mine for many years — one of my favorites. A few gray hairs emerged on her muzzle a little earlier than I would have expected, a reflection perhaps of her trauma. Only a few things reminded us of those three long months. The wrist on her right leg didn't bend quite as much as the left. A little scar from the surgery site decorated the inside of her leg like a tattoo. On cold mornings there was a little more stiffness when she first woke up. And whenever she saw me, there was always that special greeting, the unmistakable look of ardor in her eyes, the gentle tugging on my hand with soft teeth, and the unique connection between special friends. Megan was my girlfriend. Just don't tell Cynthia!

Mrs. Garner and her mother were the proud companions of a lovely little Boston terrier named Mischief. Mischief was young, only about five years old, and was aptly named, given her penchant for always finding the perfect way to cause unmitigated consternation to her besotted owners. I had treated her through many bouts of gastrointestinal distress after she had consumed some offensive inedible she had found in the yard. Fortunately, she had always responded beautifully to these treatments and had bounced right back to her normal trouble-seeking self.

When I noticed Mischief's name on the appointment book early one morning, I suspected another round of the same. But as soon as I entered the exam room, I knew this was a problem on a different order of magnitude. I could see it reflected on the faces of Mrs. Garner and her elderly mother; their faces were drawn and tense, their lips thin and tight with worry.

One look at Mischief and I knew that she was in danger. She, too, was tense and dull, her eyes cast in shadow and her short coiled tail still. For a moment she rallied when I entered the room, her tail making tiny circles and her face becoming animated. But before I could even respond to her, she was quiet again and panting heavily. Even that small an exertion had exhausted her.

"My goodness, Mischief is not feeling like herself at all, is she?" I asked, concerned.

"Not at all," responded the elderly woman, her face etched with fear. "She's been getting worse and worse over the last two days. Honestly, Dr. Coston, I don't think she's going to make it. Don't you think we should just put her down? I hate to see her suffer."

"I think it's way too early to be making any decisions like that. I haven't even examined her yet. When did all this start?"

"I first noticed her not feeling well maybe four or five days ago. I thought at the time it was probably the same old thing, so I didn't worry too much about it. But it just kept getting worse. Now she won't eat and is as weak as a dishrag."

"Let's take a look, why don't we. Put her up on the table."

Mrs. Garner lifted her onto the tabletop, where Mischief hunkered down, sad-eyed and submissive, bereft of any mischief at all. Having treated Mischief since puppyhood, I knew this lack of interest was foreign to her.

Every veterinarian develops his own systematic approach to examining a patient. This routine keeps one focused on the whole patient, rather than on just the most obvious problem. Such a comprehensive look has often saved me from making diagnostic mistakes that might have had life-threatening consequences. For me, this routine starts at the head. I examine the eyes and nose, then the mouth. From there, I feel the lymph nodes before listening carefully to the heart and the lungs with my stethoscope. I then turn my attention to the abdomen, probing with my fingers till I have felt the kidneys, the liver, the spleen, the bladder, and the intestines. I finish the examination by looking carefully at the skin and finally the musculoskeletal and nervous systems. It is important to perform the physical examination carefully on every patient, not being distracted from any part of it just because the problem seems immediately obvious. The additional information gleaned from a complete evaluation is often of vital importance.

Habits though, like rules, are made to be broken. And if there was ever a case where a problem seemed obvious upon initial evaluation, it was Mischief's. As I lifted her lip and looked in her mouth, the sheer pallor of the oral tissues shocked me. So white were they that when I tried to blanch them by pressing on them with my finger to see how quickly the color would return, there was no discernible difference in the color of the gums. Mischief was terribly anemic. The remainder of my physical examination protocol was aborted as I whisked her away to collect blood for testing.

The results of the tests were just as alarming as the lack of color on her gums. The hematocrit, a measure of the red cell mass, was only 9 percent. It should have been at least 35 percent or so. Mischief had less than one-third of the red cells she needed to carry oxygen to her body — a level that, if it dropped any lower, would be fatal. Mischief's condition was critical!

In this situation, it is the job of the clinician to identify the cause of this drop in red blood cells as quickly as possible and to institute treatment that will reverse it. The three categories of diseases that can cause these signs include blood loss, failure of the bone marrow to produce red cells, or destruction of red blood cells. Within each of these broad categories are a number of discrete causes, but getting to the correct category is the doctor's first priority.

Blood loss is relatively easy to rule out. Since there were no external wounds on Mischief that were actively spurting blood, I needed to rule out blood loss in the gastrointestinal tract. This would show up in the colon as either bright red blood, if the bleeding was in the lower GI tract, or black and tarry stool if the blood loss was in the upper GI tract.

I pulled a glove out of the drawer below the examination table and pulled it on with a smart snapping of the latex at the wrist, a sound that usually evokes an emotional response from either the patient or the owner, and often both. The truth is, nothing pleasant can ever happen for a patient of any species after a doctor puts on a glove. Some orifice is about to be probed or some bodily fluid is about to be forfeited, against the wishes of the donor. These procedures are generally not consensual. In Mischief's case, however, it was unavoidable. The normal-appearing stool on the finger of the glove ruled out blood loss as a cause of her anemia.

Red-cell production is measured by evaluating the number of immature red blood cells, called reticulocytes, which are present in the bloodstream. If the reticulocyte count is elevated, then it's obvious that the bone marrow is doing its job at peak capacity. Mischief's reticulocyte count had skyrocketed into the range where lack of red-cell production was inconceivable. That left only the category of red-cell destruction as the cause of her anemia.

This was not a surprise to me. In dogs of Mischief's age, a condition called immune-mediated hemolytic anemia (IMHA) is by far the most common cause of profound anemia. IMHA is a disease that incites the immune system to turn the full brunt of its fury against a dog's own red blood cells, destroying them with amazing ferocity and speed. On more than one occasion, I have helplessly watched with horror as a patient's red-cell count dropped by half in the span of only three or four hours. It is a nail-biting race to see if powerful drugs with awful side effects can stop the carnage before too many of the red cells are wiped out. Some races are won, but all too many of these cases end in sadness.

The vast majority of IMHA cases are categorized as idiopathic. This is a word that few of my clients are familiar with. I describe it to them as meaning that none of us idiots can figure it out; and while that description may occasionally be an accurate one, technically it means that no specific cause can be found. So *idiopathic* has come to represent a category of diseases that just happen without apparent cause — unfortunate accidents of metabolism or malicious chance. While I usually look to find a cause for IMHA, seldom do I identify one — a reality that after many years can incite complacency for the search.

I had suspected IMHA the moment I lifted Mischief's lip, and the results of the diagnostic tests had confirmed it. Given the invariably poor prognosis listed in all the veterinary textbooks and my own personal history with cases such as this, I was worried for Mischief. I gave Mrs. Garner and her mother a very guarded prognosis for her recovery.

When I laid out the odds for recovery and the treatment that would be required, they were quite reluctant to proceed, leaning instead toward a very difficult and irreversible decision. I encouraged them to stand firm and give the medication a day or two to work before giving up. But despite the encouragement I offered, I was none too confident about the outcome. With as much optimism as I could muster, I placed an intravenous catheter into her leg and began to pour a pharmacopoeia of drugs into her weakened system, hoping against hope that they would halt the red-cell destruction.

I fretted about Mischief all morning and into the early afternoon, pulling a tiny blood sample every hour to see if the red-cell count was dropping even lower or if the medications I was streaming into her were working. With intense interest, I watched her attitude to see if I could catch even a hint of a rally.

What it was that got me to go back and finish my aborted physical examination, I can no longer remember. I suspect it was the nagging suspicion that there was something I had missed that might give me the edge over such a formidable foe. So early in the afternoon, with no appreciable improvement in Mischief's condition, I put her on the exam table again. This time my examination was slow and exhaustive. Even so, I came up with no additional information. Frustrated, I started again at her head and went through the process a second time. This time I was surprised to feel something slip through my fingers as I felt the abdominal cavity, an unexpected finding in the area of the stomach. I rushed her to the X-ray room for a quick picture.

As I slapped the developed film onto the lighted view box, I was surprised to see the outline of something odd in the stomach. I couldn't identify exactly what it was, but it was obviously foreign, clearly metallic, and had the appearance of a little Oriental pagoda. In an instant of clarity as I looked at that X-ray, it all made sense. I knew with certainty that the foreign body was leaching trace amounts of a toxic heavy metal, which was causing the destruction of the red cells. I didn't know yet exactly what the metal was, but I realized that this was the cause of all Mischief's problems. That metal had to come out!

This conclusion was easier to reach than to accomplish, however. Mischief, in her current state, was anything but a good surgical candidate. But I also knew that until that foreign body was gone, she would not improve. Of that, I was convinced.

I called Mrs. Garner and described the situation in as much detail as possible. The surgery would be dicey, not because it would be a particularly difficult one but because Mischief's profound anemia made her a tenuous patient. While there was a chance we would lose her during the procedure, there was no chance of recovery without it. And if we were successful, Mischief's odds of complete recovery were excellent. After taking some time to discuss it with her mother, Mrs. Garner called back and gave me permission to proceed.

I immediately began to drip a transfusion of fresh blood into Mischief's catheter as we prepared for the surgery. Within an hour or so, I was making my first incision through Mischief's skin, holding my breath as I did so. It was a relatively simply thing to locate the stomach, make a quick incision through the pale wall, and fish out the heavy foreign body, which had sunk into the depths of the flaccid organ. What I pulled out was a stack of coins joined together by the sticky stomach contents: two quarters, two dimes, a nickel, and a penny — seventy-six cents worth of misery, illness, worry, and pain.

After closing the incision in the stomach, flushing the abdominal cavity with warm sterile saline, and placing a neat row of symmetrical stitches in Mischief's skin, I examined the coins carefully. The pagoda shape I had seen on the X-rays was explained by the way the coins had stacked up on themselves in the stomach: both quarters, then a dime, then the nickel, another dime, and finally the penny. The quarters, dimes, and nickel appeared pristine, as if they had just been cleaned with a ring cleaner. But the penny had turned a strange dark color, almost black, and had a hole eaten completely through its center.

In 1982, as a cost-saving measure, the composition of pennies changed from 95 percent copper to 97.5 percent zinc with a thin overlay of copper. While this change has saved the government millions in precious metals, it has cost pet owners a considerable sum in veterinary bills. For some reason, stray change seems to be an irresistible treat for young dogs and cats, who gulp them down like hard candy. In the stomach, the thin copper layer of the penny is eaten away by the stomach acid. Because other coins are made of other metals, they do not suffer the same fate. This would be only a cosmetic issue for the penny, if not for the zinc underneath. The effect of zinc toxicity is to create a cascade of red-blood cell destruction, which presents as the quintessential case of IMHA.

This is what had occurred in Mischief. After the coins were removed from her stomach, her recovery was rapid and complete. Two weeks after the surgery, at the time of the suture removal, her red-cell count had climbed back to normal and she was back to her mischievous ways. It was a joy to lift her lip and see the healthy glow of pinkness rush immediately back after I blanched the tissues with my finger. This, though, was hard to do with Mischief snorting and squirming and nipping playfully at my fingers. Her uninterested, dull demeanor seemed a distant memory. As I turned her on her side to remove the stitches from her shaved tummy, she wriggled and writhed in absolute glee, her short tail twisting in tight circles and her entire back end wagging excitedly.

"Wow, this is a different dog from the one you brought in two weeks ago!" I exclaimed with pleasure.

"You are so right. She's completely back to her old self now. We can't tell you how grateful we are to you. You saved her life."

"I'm just glad you brought her in when you did. I don't think she would have survived if you had waited any longer."

"Now, I'm not complaining about the bill or anything, Dr. Coston," Mrs. Garner said apologetically. "I know these things cost money. And I know how much more it would have been if I had had the same procedures done on myself. Mom just had a minor procedure done on an outpatient basis and it was way more than Mischief's whole abdominal exploratory."

It's true. Veterinary medicine remains the best bargain in any branch of health care. Veterinarians appreciate the necessity of keeping costs as low as possible for pet owners, and we generally have done a great job of that. Procedures on our patients, for which we charge a few hundred dollars, easily cost tens of thousands in a human hospital. We veterinarians have the paradoxical luxury that the actual costs of medical decisions are borne by the ones who are making them for their beloved pet. This, unfortunately, forces loving pet owners to sometimes make heart-wrenching decisions on the basis of those costs. But it has also forced veterinarians to maintain tight controls on costs and fees, a necessity that no doubt would have protected the human health-care field from the current fiscal stresses upon it. In this area, human physicians could learn much from their veterinary counterparts.

"We'd have paid anything to get Mischief back to health again. But it sure did set us back." Mrs. Garner chuckled and gave me a good-natured shake of her head.

"I know the treatment was expensive, Mrs. Garner," I said sympathetically. "But Mischief did do something that no other patient has ever done in all my years of practice."

The two turned to me expectantly. "What was that?"

"Seventy-six cents may not be much, but she's the first patient that has contributed cash to help pay the bill."

SNAKEBITE

I was delighted to see Megan dragging Elaine into the lobby of the hospital one warm late-summer morning. Though it had been a couple of years since her injury, Megan's attachment to me had not flagged. She still came in the door each time looking for me, calling out to me with a little *boof,* ears erect as she listened for my response. Megan and Elaine, though, were not alone this particular morning. Max limped in behind them, completely devoid of Megan's eagerness.

"Megan!" I said loudly. "How's my girl?"

This greeting threw her into spasms of delight, her mouth wide and laughing as she strained against the leash. Elaine released the leather handle and Megan launched herself at me, vaulting onto the reception desk between us. I met her at its summit, to find my face slathered without apology by Megan's licking tongue. It's nice to be worshiped, to be viewed by another as wonderful, heroic, handsome, and worthy. Though I had been the one who had put her through the intense discomfort of treating her badly mangled leg, this is exactly how Megan saw me still. And it was flattering! I indulged in this completely unwarranted devotion shamelessly.

When we could finally dislodge Megan from the desktop and settle her enthusiasm, I recognized the reason for today's visit. Max hunkered down behind Elaine, head low and tail between his legs, holding up one grisly front paw. He looked very much like Megan. Both had been adopted from a local shelter within a month or two of each other. As far as Ms. Farmer knew, there was no relation between them. But you would have expected them to be siblings, so similar were their markings, size, and features. Like Megan's, Max's nose was long and straight as a collie's. He, too, was longhaired and brown, though shaded with deeper reds. Like her, he was lean and had a deep, narrow chest. But that's where the similarities stopped. Max's personality was much more reserved than his infatuated sister's. Instead of incessantly seeking attention, he was more inclined to hide behind Megan or Elaine and act as if I was not present. Apparently, he had plenty of friends and felt no need to make more, especially one dressed in a white smock with a stethoscope around his neck and, God forbid, a thermometer in his hand.

Though he didn't want me to see him, it was clear that he needed my attention. His left front leg was swollen from the elbow to the toes to three or four times its normal size. The skin was darkened from a strawberry red at the top to almost a plum purple color near the foot. The twin trails of dark blood that seeped from two small punctures on the inside of the leg, at which Max licked incessantly, made the diagnosis obvious. Snakebite!

"How long has Max's leg been like that, Elaine?" I asked, concerned.

"Well, I didn't think much about it at first. He came home two nights ago limping some. By yesterday morning it was pretty swollen. But it got really bad throughout the day yesterday, and I knew I had to bring him in this morning. It's a snakebite, isn't it?"

In Virginia we have two species of poisonous snakes, water moccasins and rattlesnakes. A bite from either can result in serious tissue damage. The consequences of a snakebite do not allow one to distinguish between the types of snakes. Neither did the location in which Ms. Farmer's home was situated. Both species could be found in the Fort. So I wasn't sure which kind of bite I was treating. In as rural a setting as that in which I practice, I have always been surprised that I don't treat more snakebites. Because they are quite uncommon, though, I do not keep the extremely expensive antivenin on hand to treat them. Antivenin works best when it's started soon after a bite, anyway. I knew it would have little effect if started this late. Fortunately, snakebites are not usually life-threatening problems.

Max's temperature was elevated from the severe inflammatory response his body had mounted. He was dull and lethargic, and his leg was extremely tender to the touch. Even the slightest pressure of my probing fingers evoked from him a quiet whine of pain and a feeble attempt to wrest his hurting leg from my grasp. But, though he clearly was suffering intensely, he remained ever the gentleman, turning his head away from me in resigned submission, rather than challenging me, as many dogs would have done.

Treating snakebite patients in the absence of antivenin is a symptomatic endeavor. The pain is relieved with powerful drugs. Shock is countered with high doses of intravenous fluids and anti-inflammatory medications. Secondary infections are prevented with antibiotics. Hot and cold soaks help to reduce swelling and local tissue damage. Sometimes even these measures fail to combat the mounting pressure from the swelling, and incisions must be made in the area to release the buildup of fluids in the limb. All of these treatments were necessary for Max over the next several days.

Each day, Elaine brought Megan in to the hospital to visit her brother. They had become fast friends over the years, and she missed his presence at the house now. However those visits affected Megan, they were miraculous for Max. His ears would perk up and his nose would begin to twitch as soon as they entered the building, and he would commence to whining and nosing the cage door. After her first visit, Megan knew exactly which cage was Max's; and once she had greeted me exuberantly, she would make her way there and return his affection through the bars. Though you would think this would have made Max depressed after she left, it was amazing how much he would settle down after her visit, eating his food only after Megan and Ms. Farmer had been to see him. His attitude would remain upbeat for an hour or two before sinking down again into his discomfort.

For a while, I wondered if we were going to win the battle. But three days later, I began to notice a subtle turning of the tide in our favor. Max's attitude improved, and he showed renewed interest in his meals even before Megan's daily visit. At first the swelling simply remained unchanged from one day to the next. Then it began to subside. The intensity of the color changes in the skin began to fade. And his fever broke. When on day four he again started to bear a bit of weight on the leg, I knew that we had won. I called Elaine and told her he was ready to be discharged.

"That's wonderful, Dr. Coston. I wasn't sure we were gonna pull this one out."

"I was pretty worried for a while there myself," I responded. "But your dogs just won't give up. And with Megan encouraging him every day, he had no choice but to get better. I know he'll be glad to be home."

"I don't know about Max, but I do know Megan appreciated the chance to see you every day. She still has such a crush on you. It's unbelievable."

I chuckled dismissively. "She is a sweetie."

"I'm not kidding, Dr. Coston. If I just say

your name, Megan will go outside and try to climb into the truck. She just loves you. I'm not sure she didn't get Max bitten by that snake on purpose."

"She wouldn't do that."

"I'm pretty sure she would. You know, for weeks after her leg healed, she would go out and jump into the creek, then bark at the door of the truck, fully expecting me to take her to your office. She had that figured out. And when we didn't go, she would sulk."

"Maybe she just wanted to get away from your property. It seems to be dangerous for your dogs. First Megan's leg, and now Max's."

"What am I going to do to prevent them from getting into another dicey situation?" she asked seriously. "I can't afford any more accidents. One of these days I'm gonna lose one of them. And I really can't afford that."

"I guess you're gonna have to move!" I laughed. "Anyway, keep up the hot and cold soaks on Max's leg for another three or four days. And try to keep him off of it as much as you can. It will take a week or longer for the bruising to go away completely. But I do expect him to recover fully. We're lucky, you know."

I watched Elaine and her two dogs make their way out the door and head to the pickup truck, Max limping noticeably on his left front leg and Megan limping just barely on the right. What a grand sight it was to see both dogs walking. One had nearly lost her leg to a vehicle, the other to a venomous snake. Both of them, I noted with pride, owed their ability to walk at all to the care we had provided. With a feeling of satisfaction, I watched Elaine assist the pair into the truck.

But I couldn't squelch the nagging thought that played unwelcomed at the fringes of my mind as I indulged this moment of satisfaction. I didn't even want to acknowledge its presence or give voice to the ridiculous notion. But neither could I quite fend it off. It was just an old wives' tale, after all, that said bad luck always comes in threes. And Max's snakebite had only been Ms. Farmer's second.

SHORTNESS OF BREATH

I watched with interest as Lisa deftly slipped a tiny intravenous catheter into the thin blue line that was the shrunken, dehydrated cephalic vein in the front leg of a three-pound kitten. Her success in performing this task would doubtless mean the difference between life and death for this gravely ill patient. I marveled at the skill she displayed with this impossibly difficult chore.

For just a moment I allowed myself to consider the path Lisa had charted over the preceding several years. Somehow she had navigated the desperate waters of grief after her husband, Steve, passed two years before. Steve had suffered burns over 70 percent of his body after a terrible accident. After cleaning his paintbrushes and rollers with paint thinner, he had gone home and stocked the fireplace. Vestiges of the paint thinner on his sleeve had ignited, and he had not been able to extinguish the flames before his upper body had sustained serious injury.

Steve had lingered for over a week in the burn unit at the University of Virginia teaching hospital in Charlottesville before finally succumbing. Lisa had become a single mother and widow before the age of thirty-five.

But in the time since that tragedy, Lisa had managed to find love again with a neighbor who had befriended her after the loss. Dave had known loss himself, having buried his wife, whom ovarian cancer had claimed much too young. Dave knew like few others the depth and breadth of Lisa's sorrow. They had shared a common bond, finding comfort in the circle of those who had overcome unthinkable sadness. Their bond had grown into much more — a sincere love and an abiding trust in each other that was born of shared and satisfied emotional needs. I had watched Lisa's mourning turn to morning again, little by little, her heart dawning new and fresh under Dave's care.

Dave had not been inattentive to Melanie and Steven junior, either. The concern he had shown for them had, with time, allowed them freedom to place their father's death into perspective. Both had matured into successful young adults. Melanie engaged her interests in fashion by becoming a costume designer for the Wayside Theater, a local live-theater company. Cynthia and I occasionally saw her there when we attended the company's productions. Steven joined the military after high school to pursue his interest in aviation. The enforced discipline of the armed services gave him needed structure and confidence. Dave became for them a steady and positive influence.

Lisa's skills were invaluable to me now in the practice. Time and again, her ever-widening inventory of clinical experience and techniques had provided just the thing needed to save a patient's life, as was the case with this kitten. Because she grew to anticipate my every therapeutic move and diagnostic thought, she made my work simple and efficient. Her remarkable ability to connect with the patients put them at ease and allowed her to do even the most uncomfortable procedure with little restraint. And for those patients who would not be calmed, she was the best restrainer I could imagine, able to keep the meanest dog or the most fractious cat still enough for me to inject a cocktail of calming sedatives into their veins.

There was now little of the old Lisa left. Gone was the insecure, unsure girl who had first begun working for me six or seven years before. No longer were her interactions ingratiating and apologetic. She had earned for herself, through effort and commitment, success and accomplishment, the most coveted of respect: her own. On the heels of that, the respect of others followed naturally. Lisa's evolution confirmed the observation that you reap what you sow. Plant the seeds of success and you will harvest success, achievement building upon achievement, accomplishment upon accomplishment. And the converse, of course, is also true. Invest nothing and your return will be nothing. Failure, too, is cumulative. Lisa had worked for these gains, and it was a wonderful thing to see the results etched into her self-assured face, her easy smile, her proficient clinical expertise.

My reverie was interrupted as Lisa finished taping the intravenous catheter in place and turned to me.

"What rate of fluids do you want this kitten to have?" she asked, then erupted with a deep and coarse cough. It took her a little while to regain her composure before she addressed me again. "Wow, I can't seem to shake this cold."

"How long have you been coughing like that?"

"Oh, it started probably a month ago or so. It's a real hanger-oner. At least I haven't been all stuffed up."

"You know what I'm going to say now, don't you?"

"Yeah, I know. I gotta give up the old cancer sticks." Lisa laughed. I had been giving her good-natured grief about her smoking for years, ever since she started working for me, in fact. But smoking was a given among her family members. All of them, including now Steven and Melanie, smoked constantly. It was a habit I simply did not understand, not ever having been tempted to start.

Two or three days later, I came upon Lisa, who was standing uncharacteristically still at the top of the stairs. She was breathing hard.

"You all right?" I asked. "You look like you just finished a marathon."

"It's really strange," she replied, laughing, "but that's just how I feel. I've gotten so completely out of shape, it takes my breath away just to come up the stairs. I gotta start exercising more. Dave and I have talked about starting to jog in the evenings, but I just can't muster the energy."

"I don't know, Lisa. With that cough and this shortness of breath, I might go see a doctor. Maybe you have a touch of bronchitis and need some antibiotics or something. No cough should go on for that long."

In my case, the stresses of veterinary school manifested as shortness of breath. It was awful: the tugging to breathe, the refusal of my lungs to expand fully, the unsuccessful attempts to suck in a full complement of oxygen. I had gone to the doctor, fearing some awful malady, and had watched him write "SOB" on my record, insulted that he thought so poorly of me. He had assured me, though, that SOB was the medical abbreviation for shortness of breath. After finding nothing amiss, he had suggested that the shortness of breath might be a consequence of the stresses and pressures of veterinary school. I had thought the suggestion ridiculous, but I was surprised when the symptoms magically and immediately resolved, not from medical intervention but from a simple psychological response to being named. So I had real empathy for Lisa's symptoms. I was sure hers would resolve, too, with a little medical attention. She had certainly been under a constant barrage of stress over the last couple of years.

"I've been thinking I ought to get checked out. I'll make an appointment soon."

That was the last I thought of it for a while. I did notice with concern that Lisa's cough did not go away and that she avoided stairs and physical exertion as much as possible. But it wasn't till about three weeks later that Lisa mentioned anything more about it.

"I went to the doctor yesterday."

"Oh yeah? What did he say?"

"He didn't think it was bronchitis, but he put me on some antibiotics just in case. He was a little concerned about walking pneumonia, so he sent me over to the hospital to get X-rays taken. I get the results of those back in a day or two. He said he'd call me."

"I'm glad you got looked at, anyway. I hope you get to feeling better."

"That's just the thing," she said. "I feel just fine." While this should have made me feel good, somehow it did just the opposite.

"Oh, and by the way," she added, "he wants me to quit smoking."

"Good man."

In the back of my mind, the details of this situation were not settling well. A bothersome, wholly unsubstantiated worry nagged at my mind. Why would Lisa be coughing and having significant shortness of breath with the slightest physical exertion but not feel at all ill? But Lisa was young and in good health, and she had certainly been under enormous pressure recently. There was no reason to suspect the worst. Besides, I was not a physician and had no business considering potential diagnoses for her. I pushed the concern from my mind.

A few days later, though, Lisa was called to the phone. I watched from the corner of my eye. The call clearly caused her some concern. After a few minutes, she came to me, obviously upset.

"Doc, the nurse from my doctor's office called. They got the results from the chest X-rays back. They want me to go to the office to discuss the results with the doctor. She said it was important that we set it up as soon as possible. They want me to go in this afternoon."

"That sounds like no fun."

"I gotta say, it's got me a little spooked." She chuckled wryly. "Anyway, I'm gonna have to be gone for a little while. Is that okay?"

"Of course. You do what you need to do. We'll get by."

When she returned to the office an hour or so later, I detected no relief on her face. In fact, she looked even more worried. She was carrying a large X-ray envelope in her hand and she motioned for me to follow her into an exam room, where she removed a large film from the envelope and placed it up on the lighted view box. X-rays of humans appear very strange to me. I am so accustomed to seeing the chest films of dogs and cats that the same views of people appear clumsily oversized and eerily distorted to gigantic proportions, like the seedy sideshows at the fair. But there are also enough similarities that I can recognize when things are amiss. Looking at Lisa's film, my eyes immediately went to an area of excessive whiteness in the lung fields, where I was sure it should have been much darker. I felt a knot tighten in my stomach.

"So what do you think?" she asked. It was flattering that my opinion mattered to her. I knew she respected my medical expertise. But this was completely outside my field of study and certainly represented dangerous emotional ground for me. The last thing I wanted to do was offer any medical opinion in areas I was not trained in, particularly regarding someone about whom I cared so much. I dodged.

"What did the doctor say?"

"He is concerned about that spot right there." She pointed to the area that had caught my eye. "He isn't sure what it is yet. So he has referred me to a respiratory specialist in Winchester. I'm supposed to go tomorrow and take the X-rays with me." She was quiet for a while, studying first the film, then my face. Then she addressed me again.

"So what do you think?"

"I think you need to do exactly what he says. There's no way to know precisely what that is without following a diagnostic path. That's why he's referring you to someone else to take the next step. And that's just what you should do." I turned from the film to face her. "It's a little disconcerting, though, isn't it? You doing okay?"

"We'll see. It does have me pretty scared, though."

"I don't blame you. But, remember, it could be anything — perhaps scar tissue or an inflammatory nodule. Some people even have lesions that show up on X-rays and look bad, but end up being aberrant heartworms. I know it's a scary thing to think the worst. But it doesn't have to be bad. It could be something simple. Let's let the doctors do their work."

And the doctors did do their work over the next several weeks. The respiratory specialist took one look at the X-rays and ordered an MRI, which showed the same lesion in more detail. The devil was in the details. Not only did it confirm the original nodule, but it also highlighted several additional areas of concern. The next step was a needle biopsy, followed by a few incredibly frightening days of waiting for those results. When the doctor's office finally called, Lisa was again in my office.

"Doc, they've called to let me know they have the results of the biopsy back." Her voice was even, but her face was strained and taut.

"What did they say?"

"They want me to go in tomorrow to discuss the results."

My stomach lurched and I could sense the sudden taste of fear in my mouth. Good news is shared over the phone by the nurse. Bad news is discussed face-to-face with the doctor. This was not what I had hoped for. Lisa knew it, too. I could see it reflected in the drawn lines on her face and the set of her mouth. I tried to downplay the significance.

"Okay, that could mean a lot of things. No —"

"Don't try to fool me, Doc," Lisa interrupted. "You know as well as I do that it probably isn't good news. Besides, they told me they have forwarded the information to an oncologist. My appointment is with the oncologist. I'm really scared now."

I leaned forward and took her hands in mine. "I know. Me, too."

"I'd really appreciate it if you'd go with me to the appointment. I'm going to have Susan go, too. I don't really have anyone else to go through this with, you know."

My mind teetered. Of course I would support her in any way I could. But this request, as much as it affirmed our friendship, pushed me far out of my comfort zone. I expected that the news the doctor had to share with Lisa was intensely personal and would have deeply intimate repercussions. The situation demanded a level of trust and personal vulnerability that took me off guard. It also frightened me. I realized that I could have difficult conversations with my clients about their beloved pets and do it with compassion, sensitivity, and tact, but to think that I might be involved in a life-and-death discussion about a person seemed more than I was prepared for.

"I'll be glad to go with you and Susan," I replied. Susan had known Lisa as long as I had. "But, Lisa, you do have someone who will be glad to stand by your side whatever the doctor says, you know. Dave will be there for you."

"I know, Doc. But this is like déjà vu for him. It hasn't been that long since he lost his wife. I don't want him to have to face this again."

The car trip to Winchester the next day was odd, the three of us riding along, trying hard to avoid the topic that was dominating our thoughts. I felt like a voyeur, peeking through private windows.

"Lisa, I need to know just what it is you want me to do at this appointment today. Do you want me to ask all the questions? Do you want me to push for details? Or do you want me just to listen and be there for you?" Susan had recently lost her mother to cancer, so I knew she was experienced at this process. She could either be the friendly shoulder for support or she could be an information gatherer. But I had no experience in this at all. I was a complete novice, and an intimidated one at that.

"Just be there and listen. Ask any questions that you think need to be asked and might get missed," she responded. "I just know this might be pretty hard for me. And in the emotion of the moment, I may not completely process or remember all the information he gives me."

We sat for a few minutes in the waiting

room. There were very few places in the world I would have wanted to be in less than the waiting room of this oncologist's office. It's not like a pediatrician's office, where most patients are perfect and full of endless possibilities. The patients here were older and appeared unfit. The room reverberated with illness and the imminence of death. Every person there, whether the patient or a loved one, vibrated with it, lived within its shroud, wore its presence like a cloak, heavy, dark, and stifling. Lisa was by far the youngest person in the room, and she looked the healthiest.

One man, who appeared to be in his mid-fifties, shuffled stiffly in and dropped uncomfortably into a chair, wincing as he did so. A woman, who I assumed was his wife, followed him, pushing a cart that held a green oxygen tank from which six feet of transparent tubing emerged, making a loop around the man's head and pumping oxygen into his nostrils. His grayish yellow skin hung loosely on him, like the fading draperies of an outdated home that had been decorated poorly. The effort of the walk into the office was evident in the loud wheezing rush of air through his open mouth and the staccato rate at which his chest heaved, punctuated by his desperate facial expression. It was as if there had been a run on the oxygen bank and he could no longer access his account. I did not want to look, but I could not pull my eyes away.

A crisp nurse in an aseptic uniform called Lisa's name, and the three of us ambled through the door, which she held open for us, smiling incongruously. I could feel the eyes of the others in the waiting room follow us; could feel their pity accompany us down the hall, squeezing through the door as it closed behind us. In the examination room, Lisa sat on the padded, paper-covered exam table, and Susan sat down on the one chair provided. I leaned against the wall until the door opened again and another chair was pushed through by the nurse. We spoke for a minute in hushed whispers, until we heard the doctor slide Lisa's medical records and X-rays out of a pocket on the other side of the door. There was a slight delay as he scanned the records for a name before pushing the door open and whisking into the room, all smiles.

"Good afternoon, Lisa," he said, extending a hand to Susan. "I'm Dr. Carver."

"Hello," Susan responded, pointing to Lisa. "That's Lisa over there."

Dr. Carver seemed surprised that his patient was clearly the youngest one in the room. "Pardon me." He laughed easily, turning to Lisa. "Your respiratory doc sent over the films, the MRI, and the biopsy results. I've had a chance to go over all of them. Unfortunately, the biopsy confirms lung cancer."

He paused and gave Lisa a moment to appropriate the words fully, keeping his eyes on her face, his expression professional, calm, and empathetic. He had clearly done this before, and he was good at it. Lisa's shoulders dropped and her breathing sped up a bit. But stoic and strong as always, she kept her eyes on Dr. Carver's face. Susan's eyes rimmed immediately with wetness, filling with tears, courage, and resolution, just the things she knew Lisa would need. Her hand went to Lisa's shoulder. Lisa did not say anything, so Dr. Carver continued.

"There are two common kinds of tumors that affect the lungs — large-cell and small-cell carcinomas. The biopsy shows that this is the small-cell variety. Unfortunately, this type generally carries the worse prognosis. It tends to be a little more aggressive and a little less responsive to chemotherapy." The news settled heavily in the room, silence wrapping each of us in our own thoughts. Dr. Carver broke the somber silence. He sat forward briskly and wrapped his locked hands around one knee, pulling it up as he leaned back again.

"That's the bad news. But we don't want to dwell on the bad parts." He hurried on, knowing, I'm sure, that the bad parts would consume all our attention anyway. "The fact is, this cancer is treatable. There are a lot of things we can do to keep it at bay. And we're going to get started right away. Now, I know I've hit you pretty hard already. I'm sure you have a million questions. So fire away."

Lisa continued to look at him, but I could tell her mind was far away in dark places. Susan took the helm.

"You said the cancer was treatable. What exactly does that mean?" she asked.

"Yes, it is treatable, though it may not be curable. With aggressive therapy, we can usually extend survival times significantly. And from the films, it appears that we've caught this pretty early."

"What kind of therapy are you talking about?" Lisa asked evenly.

"We usually use a combination protocol of several chemotherapy medications, all given intravenously. We can follow up with radiation to get the tumors as small as possible. I know chemo sounds scary, and honestly, it's no picnic. But we've come a long way in how well we're able to control side effects. Most of my patients continue to feel pretty good throughout."

"How long?" Lisa asked quietly.

"We usually start with a six-to-nine-week course of chemo. Then we'll adjust our schedule depending on response."

"No," she said. "How long are these extended survival times?"

"The research indicates that the average patient lives about a year or a year and a half with chemo. But you have to remember, that's an average. And averages are made up of some people who live much longer."

"And some who don't live as long," Lisa said.

"That's true, of course, but you have a lot of positive factors on your side. You're young and healthy. We've caught this pretty early. And you obviously have the support of some very good friends and family. Those are really important considerations."

"What causes these types of tumors?" Lisa asked.

"Are you a smoker?"

"Yeah. I've smoked since I was a teen-ager."

"That's the biggest risk factor. But here's the thing. It doesn't matter anymore what caused it. What matters now is how we go after it. I'd like you to stop smoking now, though. Do you think you can do that?"

"I don't have much choice now, do I? I'll do whatever I have to do."

"That's the spirit. It's really important for the patient to have a positive, can-do attitude about the disease and its treatment."

"Can I keep working during my treatment?"

"You can continue to do everything you feel good enough to do. Most patients end up needing to take some time off, though. They tend to get pretty nauseous and tired, and that often interferes with how much they can do. But we'll give you plenty of medicine for your tummy. What is it that you do?"

"I'm a veterinary technician. We've treated quite a few cancer patients at our clinic. Dr. Coston is my boss." Lisa nodded her head in my direction.

"Really!" Dr. Carver turned to me with interest. We spoke for a few minutes about chemotherapy in my patients, the types of cancers I saw the most, the drugs I used, the methods employed to control side effects. He was intrigued, but I felt uncomfortable with the focus turned away from Lisa. He turned again to her.

"Okay, Lisa," he said cheerfully. "I want to get you started right away. The nurse will come in and take you to our chemotherapy room in a few minutes for the first round. We're going to get through this together. Are there any other questions?"

Susan jumped in. "What kind of side effects should she expect from this?"

"The typical side effects hit one of three areas: the GI tract, with vomiting and diarrhea; the bone marrow, with low white-blood-cell counts; or the hair follicles, with hair loss. That's why you see a lot of cancer patients with shaved heads. The GI stuff we can usually control pretty well with medications. The bone marrow effects we watch pretty closely. Sometimes we need antibiotics if the white cells drop too low. Those things, we can do something about. The hair, not so much. Anything else?"

We were all quiet. This had been what we had expected, but we were stunned nonetheless. Dr. Carver stood, shook hands all around, and walked out the door. Silence settled on us like white in a snow globe. Susan turned her attention to Lisa, searching her face for clues of how she was dealing with the news. Lisa's eyes were haunted and hollow, searching the ground. Her face was drawn. She sat on her hands and rocked slowly back and forth.

For my part, I was sad, deeply so. But in

short order, I realized that I was also angry. This was just not fair! It was not fair to Lisa, who had suffered one slamming defeat after another in her short life. It was certainly not fair to Melanie and Steven, who likely would be orphans in a few months, having lost first their father to a freak accident and then their mother. It was not fair to Lisa's mother, Amelia, with whom Lisa still lived. A parent is not supposed to bury her child. It's supposed to be the other way around. How could this make sense in any way?

The reality was, however, that my anger was a wasted emotion. There just wasn't anyone to be angry at. Certainly not Lisa, though her teenage choice to smoke had most likely led her into this room. The nicotine habit had long ago taken that choice away from her, imprisoning her in a practically escape-proof psychological fortress of addiction. Besides, what Lisa needed most from me now was not anger but support. I vowed to do what I could to help her.

The nurse pushed the door open again, interrupting our private ruminations. She led us down the hall to a large room where perhaps eight or ten plush armchairs were situated in two rows. Behind each chair rose a metal pole from which was suspended a bag of medication. Every chair was filled with a patient in some degree of decline. The people sat patiently in their chairs, reading paperbacks and listening to music through headphones. Most of the chairs hummed and vibrated, their automatic massage functions working at full capacity. Nurses fluttered among the chairs like waitresses, carrying more bags of fluid from the back room, checking on patients, taking blood pressure readings, and delivering snacks and drinks.

Lisa was directed to an empty recliner, and a nurse landed in a chair next to her. Before we knew it, Lisa had a catheter in her arm and fluids running rapidly into her veins. An ominous, darkly colored bag was hung over her head and the nurse hooked its tubes into the plastic plumbing that was already flooding fluids into her. The treatment took an hour or two to complete, and then the receptionist expeditiously penned in an appointment for her next treatment. Lisa was issued a ream of prescriptions, which we needed to fill at a pharmacy. And then we were back in the car, heading home.

The news struck the office like a tornado, leaving disorganized piles of emotional debris scattered among the staff. We were a close team, and having one of our own down seemed a heavy load to bear. Cynthia was deep into the planning of our Christmas party, but the developments with Lisa took the joy out of it. The staff just could not stomach a Christmas party that year, and the plans were scrapped.

Cynthia and I gave much thought to how we could best help Lisa through the long ordeal ahead of her. The biblical injunction to help the widows and the orphans figured prominently in our discussions; Lisa and Melanie and Steven certainly fit that bill. We discussed several options, settling at last on a plan. Two days after the trip to the oncologist's office, I made my way to Lisa's house after work. Lisa and I sat down in her living room.

"Lisa, I've given this a lot of thought. I can't imagine how hard this must be for you. I know there must be a thousand things occupying your mind these days."

"You could say that."

"Here's what I want to do. I want to take as many worries away from you as I can. The doctor said when we were there that most chemo patients have to take some time off from work for their treatments."

"Yeah, I've thought about that, too. I don't want to leave you in the lurch, though. And frankly, I really need all the hours I can get

now, with all the medical bills and everything. So I don't plan on taking any more
time off than absolutely necessary."

"Here's the thing, Lisa. I don't want you
to worry about that. The office is my responsibility. As far as I'm concerned, your full-
time job right now is to get better. So I'm
going to continue to pay your full-time sal-
ary throughout your treatment. You work as
much as you're able to. But if you need to
take some time off, do what you need to do
to get well. I know you well enough to know
that you will be at the office whenever
you're able. But if you're not feeling up to
it, don't worry. You'll still get your hours."

Lisa was silent for a long time. Then I
noticed her lip beginning to quiver and her
eyes filling with tears. Lisa began to cry on
my shoulder. She cried for a long time,
emptying a full container of emotional de-
tritus that had collected over the last month
or two of X-rays, of blood tests, of MRIs,
and doctor's visits, of bad news and worse
news, of maintaining a strong facade for
Melanie and Steven and Amelia. These were
the first and last tears I saw Lisa cry over
her own illness. And when the tears finally
ceased, she seemed a bit more at ease. I left
that evening feeling confident that Lisa
knew Cynthia and I were on her side and

were cheering her on and hoping against all expectations, against all the medical literature, against even the fates that seemed once again to have lined up against her, that this time she might win; that this time Lisa's luck would hold and the cancer would shrink and shiver and shrivel up to nothing. That's all we could do — support her and hope and pray. And that's what we did.

Max's Crisis

"Looks like your girlfriend may be coming in this morning," Susan said, smiling conspiratorially, as I walked into the hospital early one Wednesday morning.

"My girlfriend?"

"Yes. Elaine Farmer has an appointment."

"Oh," I replied. "You mean my girlfriend Megan. Is there something wrong with her?"

"No. The appointment book says that we need to check Max's breathing. But Elaine usually brings Megan along when she comes, so she can see you."

I sorted through a list of reasons why Max might need to have his breathing checked. At only about six or seven years old, he was too young to be in heart failure, I thought. Usually, heart disease afflicts senior dogs. Perhaps he'd developed pneumonia or even something as mild as an upper respiratory virus. Anyway, I wouldn't have to wait long to find out. Max's appointment was fairly early in the morning. I was looking forward to seeing my girlfriend anyway.

When Elaine and Max came through the door an hour or two later, however, Megan wasn't with them. As usual, Max was not eager to come into the building, dodging instead down the handicapped ramp. With effort, Elaine tugged on the leash, finally coercing Max to enter the lobby. He immediately hunkered down under the bench seat, hiding behind Elaine's legs as soon as she sat down.

They had to wait only a few minutes before Lisa escorted them into an exam room and got Max's weight and temperature. As I finished writing the record from my previous patient, Lisa emerged from the room and handed me Max's chart.

"Something's really not right with Max," she reported, a look of dread on her face. "He's lost almost six pounds since he was here last month. And, man, is he tugging to breathe. He breathes about like me."

Elaine had on a pair of faded jeans and a light jacket. But she was also clothed with worry. It was in her eyes, the set of her jaw, and the slump of her shoulders. It filled the room; I could feel it as I entered. And it extended to my patient, as well. Whether Max had sensed it from Elaine's emotional cues or felt it himself, I wasn't sure. But there was concern and fear in his eyes, too — fear that was more than the usual anxiety about being in the hospital and being probed with a thermometer. He seemed aware that something just wasn't right.

The reason for this worry was evident right away. It didn't take a medical genius to see that Max was struggling for each breath. My immediate impression was that Max was not in heart failure. Cardiac patients have a particular presentation, one that, after so many years, I sense almost intuitively. Which subtle cue it was in Max that made me think his heart was not the problem was not immediately apparent. Perhaps it was the glint of confusion, almost panic, in his eyes as he tugged at the air, willing a little oxygen into the depths of his lungs. That was it, the sheer effort it took for Max to suck the breath into his chest — effort he exerted in his belly to suction in even the little bit he could, each attempt seeming to corral only the tiniest bit of coveted air.

Heart patients' breathing is different. While they breathe hard, too, it isn't with this same effort just to draw in the air. The act of breathing isn't the problem for a heart patient. The problem is in exchanging the oxygen taken in. Patients with lung disease breathe in a different way, too. Their difficulty is not with drawing in the air but with exhaling it. Their abdominal effort comes as they breathe out; a final squeeze with their tummies at the end of each breath to chase a little more of the air out of their diseased lungs. Max's pattern was neither of these.

As I listened to his chest, I involuntarily furrowed my brow with concentration. I would be a poor poker player. This flinching of my face is my tell to worried clients that something about their pet's case is puzzling me. Sometimes it's just a sign of the extra intensity required to hear a heart that is beating four times faster than ours that does it. But often it is because there is a murmur, a missed beat, or fluid crackling in the lungs. In Max's case, it was due to the fact that I could hear vigorous air movement in the upper portions of his lung fields, but below a line I could draw horizontally across his chest, there was nothing. I should have been able to hear air rushing through his airways down there as well, but even his pounding heart was muffled as I listened.

"You look worried," Elaine said, her own concern springing afresh to her face. "What are you hearing?"

"It's what I'm not hearing that has me concerned. I should be able to hear it all over his chest as the air moves in his lungs. But I can hear no air movement below here," I said, drawing my finger across Max's chest from front to back.

"That's not good."

"No, it's not," I agreed. "That's probably why he's working so hard to breathe. Something is preventing him from pulling a full breath.. Did this start all at once? Or did it slowly get worse and worse?"

"I honestly don't know, Dr. Coston." Elaine shook her head in confusion. "Max took off and was gone for a few days. He was fine when he left. But when he came back, he was breathing like this. So I don't know if it came on slowly over a few days or started quickly."

"Were there any signs of injury that you noticed?"

"None that I could see, though he was moving pretty slowly, now that you mention it." Elaine paused a moment, remembering back over the course of events. "So what would make it so you couldn't hear lung sounds down there?"

"Well, it could be a bunch of different things: fluid buildup, air accumulation around the lungs, a mass in the chest, or a ruptured diaphragm. We're going to need X-rays to help us sort that out."

"Do whatever you need to do. I can't stand to see him like this."

Elaine left Max with me, making me promise to call her as soon as I had any information. I took Max into the treatment room and had Lisa get blood work and take pictures of his chest as quickly as possible. Within an hour I was holding his lab results. They were normal. Whatever was causing this problem was not related to organ failure. The X-rays, hopefully, would make the diagnosis evident.

The picture that greeted me when I placed Max's chest X-rays on the lighted view box was a strange one. Where there should have been dark, air-filled lungs, I saw instead a very white pattern in the bottom half of the lung fields. Scattered throughout this white background were dark streaks of gas patterns that looked exactly like the gas seen occasionally in intestines. And the starkly contrasting curved sheet of diaphragm which normally separates the chest cavity from the abdomen was evident only in the top of the picture. Somehow Max had ruptured his diaphragm.

Two things make breathing difficult when a diaphragm is torn. First, the plunger function of this sheet of muscle tissue is lost, making it very difficult to pull air into the lungs, just as a syringe would be useless without the rubber stopper at the end of the plunger that allows negative pressure to develop within the barrel of the syringe as the plunger is pulled back. Second, liver and intestines often spill through the hole in the diaphragm and take up the space in the chest cavity normally occupied by the lungs.

This situation needed to be corrected — and fast. In these cases, a demanding surgery to repair the defect in the diaphragm is usually curative. The tricky part of this surgery is breathing for the patient when the abdominal cavity is opened, since, with the hole in the diaphragm, there can be no negative pressure generated and the lungs simply cannot fill with air on their own. This makes it necessary for the surgical team to ventilate the patient mechanically fifteen or more times each minute, forcing air into the lungs. This artificial respiration must be carefully coordinated with the work of the surgeon, who, between each hand-pumped breath, must return all the abdominal organs to their normal positions and sew the huge hole in the diaphragm closed, creating a tight seal and leaving no leaks. For the surgeon, coordinating all these intricate details is like directing a symphony.

I called Ms. Farmer and outlined the diagnosis and the surgery that would need to be done in order to correct the condition. She, as always, calmly took the information in stride.

"What do you think caused the diaphragm to tear?"

"It's usually a traumatic event. If I was a betting man, I'd say that Max got bumped by a car during the time he was gone."

"That makes sense. Maybe that's why it took him so long to make his way home."

"I'm sure you're right."

"When will you do the surgery?"

"I think it needs to be done right away. My staff is already clearing my schedule. As soon as we have a catheter in place and get the surgery suite set up, we'll get right on it."

"Okay," she replied. "I have absolute confidence in you. Do what you need to do. Remember, Max is very important to me. I know I may lose him, but do your best. That's all I ask."

It is always with a deep respect, an overwhelming sense of awe, and a keen awareness of the importance of each patient that I embark upon the task of treating a beloved pet. This feeling is magnified when I do surgery, especially a challenging one like the repair of a diaphragmatic hernia. But when a client sets the stage for a procedure as Elaine had, the pressure upon me to perform at my peak is so much the greater. I knew exactly what I needed to do and had done it many times before, but it was with an extra degree of nervous energy that I paused with my scalpel above Max's belly that day. Bolstered by Elaine's vote of confidence, I made a bold incision.

What I found was not a surprise. About a third of Max's liver had found its way into his chest cavity. Part of the spleen and a few loops of bowel had followed. It was a simple thing to pull these back into his abdomen. I could watch, through the gaping hole in the diaphragm, the pink lungs fill with air as the assistant squeezed the breathing bag. I could see how much easier they were able to fill. And I could see the heart beating vigorously inside the pericardial sac and could feel its vitality with my gloved finger. The edges of the rent in the diaphragm were pulled together with strong sutures, by my placing the needle through the muscle tissues carefully between breaths. After tying the last knot in the suture line on the diaphragm, I tested the seal by inflating the lungs to capacity with the breathing bag and listening for bubbles to escape through the suture line. There were none — no leaks. What remained was to place a tube into the chest cavity. The tube exited through the skin; it allowed me to evacuate the residual air around the lungs and any blood or fluids that might accumulate. Finally, I closed the abdominal wall and sutured the skin.

The surgery had taken over two hours to complete and I was drained. But Max was recovering nicely and already breathing more easily. I was pleased with the day's work. As promised, I called Elaine and reported that the surgery was over and had been successful. I expected to keep Max in the hospital for at least two days, until the amount of material sucked from the tube in his chest had subsided enough to allow its removal.

Elaine brought Megan in to visit Max and me on Friday. While it was wonderful to see her, the effect on Max was not what I expected. Instead of perking him up, Megan's visit seemed to increase his stress, shooting his respiratory rate up and tiring him noticeably.

The day after surgery I was able to remove a few milliliters of fluid and a couple of syringefuls of air from Max's chest. By that Friday, the amount had decreased even more. Even so, Max was not bouncing back as quickly as I had expected him to. I decided that he needed continued care over the weekend, and I told Elaine I thought he should stay with me. She seemed relieved.

When I came in to the hospital on Saturday morning, I found Max's breathing to be labored again. What worried me just as much was the look of anxiety that had crept back onto his face. I suspected air or fluid was leaking into the chest cavity. But when I aspirated the tube with the syringe, nothing came out. I needed X-rays to evaluate the problem, and I needed help to take them. Fortunately, Susan was willing to come from home to assist me.

When, in less than an hour, I was once again placing Max's chest X-rays up on the view box, I was shocked to see a pattern almost identical to the films I had taken before surgery. There was the same light density at the bottom of the film, the same intestinal gas pattern where it shouldn't have been, the same discontinuity to the diaphragmatic shadow.

"Oh no," I said, letting out a deep sigh. "It looks like the whole incision line in the diaphragm has broken down. We're going to have to go back in."

"You're kidding!" Susan had enough track

record with my sense of humor to think I was pulling her leg.

"No, Susan. I wish I was kidding, but I'm not! And what's worse, I don't think it should wait till we're open again on Monday. I think we ought to do it today."

"Okay. But we will need extra help, won't we?"

"Yes. We'll need at least one more person. You can scrub in to assist me. We'll need someone to ventilate Max and monitor the anesthesia."

"Lisa's out of town, you know."

"Oh shoot," I responded. The anesthesia for a case like this was especially difficult, and Lisa was the only licensed technician at the hospital at that time. "We'll have to call in Ginny. We can walk her through the procedure beforehand. You call her and I'll call Elaine."

This was not a call I particularly relished. Ms. Farmer was expecting a routine update on Max's continuing recovery. What she was going to hear instead was that another frightening surgery was necessary. I picked up the phone with a measure of dread. But I needn't have worried. Elaine was her usual unflappable and controlled self when I told her the news.

"Well, that's not what I wanted to hear,

371

but I had a feeling things were not going as well as we wanted them to when I was in to visit him yesterday. Even Megan couldn't spark any enthusiasm. And that's not like Max at all." She paused for a moment before continuing. "Say, Dr. Coston. Would you mind if I came in and observed the surgery? I wanted to watch the first one, but I was too busy to get away. I do have time today, though."

I choked a bit on the phone, and she sensed my hesitation. "That is, if it's okay with you. I wouldn't want to go against your better judgment."

It was indeed against my better judgment to let owners observe surgeries on their pets. There had just been too many times over the years when such a plan had injected unnecessary drama into an otherwise-routine procedure. But this was different. Elaine had quite a bit of clinical experience in her work. She probably would not get queasy. She was also very educated and levelheaded. Nor did I have a great deal of high ground to stand on. This was, after all, the second time I was going to have to do surgery for the same problem. Accommodating her request, I thought, was wise, though there was still trepidation in my heart. Had she not been so magnanimous, I probably would have said no.

"Okay. If you really want to, I'll let you come. But it can be a pretty tense operation. I don't want you to be alarmed with the process — no matter what happens, okay?" But I wasn't really concerned about Elaine. She was just so self-possessed. I expected no problems from her.

Ginny arrived a few minutes later. Ginny was a short, lean woman about thirty-five years old. A no-nonsense, take-charge person, she was extremely capable and committed to doing everything just right. She had been a loyal client before approaching me for a job, timing her query just when I needed someone as an assistant. The vast array of individual tasks and the intensity and quantity of work done in the hospital had surprised her, as it does most new staff members. As she did not always feel proficient enough to perform to the level she expected of herself or at the speed she wished, this frustrated her.

I often recall with a chuckle her response to me one busy day when I added a new task to her already-long list of chores. She fixed me with a look mixed with equal parts humor and irritation and said, "Well, just stick a broom in my behind and I can sweep while I walk!"

I could see the exasperation on her face as soon as Ginny walked into the treatment room, where Susan and I were going over the materials we would need for the surgery. I knew that it was not from frustration at having to come in on a weekend. Ginny wasn't like that. It was instead concern that she would not be able to do what I asked of her. There was foreboding on her face as I outlined exactly what she would do. But when I told her that Elaine was going to come in and observe, I thought she might just kick me.

Susan and I had given Max the anesthetics through his catheter and were inserting into his airway the tube through which we would administer the anesthetic gases when Elaine arrived. Ginny escorted her into the treatment room. Quickly I secured the endotracheal tube in place by pulling it to the roof of Max's mouth and tying it around his nose and upper jaw with a length of gauze.

Susan and Ginny busied themselves scrubbing and sterilizing the surgery site. Max was laid out on his back, his front legs pulled over his head and the surgery table tilted dramatically so his head was lower than his chest. I gave Elaine a quick summary of the task at hand and what she would be seeing. I was careful to explain the process of manual ventilation, which the tear in the diaphragm made necessary. Then I began the ten-minute process of scrubbing my hands, donning a surgical gown, and pulling on a pair of sterile gloves in preparation for surgery.

Since I had completed surgery just three days previously, entering Max's abdomen again involved simply cutting and removing the sutures that had been placed at that time and separating the already-healing tissues. Once I had entered the abdomen, I was surprised at what I found. I was not surprised that there was a diaphragmatic hernia. The surprise was to find that the liver, part of the spleen, and the intestines were bulging into the chest cavity not on the right side as they had been before, but through a hole that was just as big on the opposite side. This shocked me so much that I double-checked myself by looking for the suture line I had placed previously. There it was, intact and holding strong.

Apparently, the initial injury had resulted in a tear in the diaphragm on not just one side but both. The abdominal organs, however, had fallen through only the tear on the right side, the one I originally found. When I had tested the diaphragm for leaks during the first surgery, the liver must have fallen against the second hole, in effect sealing any leakage through it during the test. The second hole had remained undetected. It was not until the second day after surgery that the liver had once again slipped through this second hole, sending Max back into respiratory distress.

The process of closing the rent in the diaphragm would have to be repeated on the other side. This was going along famously, the four of us idly sharing pleasantries as I stitched, when all of a sudden Max's heartbeat sped up noticeably and he involuntarily coughed. It is not unusual for a surgical patient's depth of anesthesia to vary a bit during the course of a procedure. This is easily managed by changing the dose of anesthetic gases administered with a quick twist of a knob on the machine. But because Max's head was tilted downward and because the gauze tied around his nose had apparently loosened during the forced ventilation, when he coughed, the tube I had inserted into his windpipe shot out like a blow dart, hitting the ground with a thud. The tubes connected to the anesthesia machine, through which passed the anesthetic gases that kept Max asleep, fell with it.

The sound made me jerk my head up from my work, my hands buried almost to the elbows in Max's deep chest. My eyes went wide, and I was immediately stricken with alarm. I noticed that Susan's eyes also registered concern. But nothing could match the ashen countenance on Ginny's panicked face. It was frozen in slack-jawed terror. The three of us knew that it was now only a matter of time before Max started waking up — and not much time at that. If he came to with both his abdomen and chest cavities open, it would be catastrophic. I could envision the scene: Max bouncing around the surgery room, intestines falling through the incision, struggling unsuccessfully for a few frantic seconds to draw air into his lungs before crumpling to the floor.

There was not a moment to lose. Jerking my hands from deep within Max's insides, I picked the tube up off the floor and ran to the sink in the next room, where I rinsed it quickly under the faucet. Then I raced back into the surgery suite, where Max was beginning to huff a bit. Standing practically on my head, I pulled his mouth open and quickly stabbed with the tube at his airway, the anatomy appearing upside down from its usual appearance because of his position on the table. Fortunately, the tube slipped easily down his trachea. Tying the gauze tightly around the tube and then again around Max's upper jaw, I secured the tube in place again before reattaching the anesthetic machine to it. The whole episode had taken less than a minute, but I was dripping with sweat and there was a noticeable ringing in my ears by the time I had finished. I could feel the blood rushing to my face, redness sweeping aside the astonishment.

My gaze made its way around the room. Ginny's eyes were wide above her surgical mask, the light blue of which contrasted sharply with the pearly white pallor of her glistening forehead. She pressed her back up against the wall, her palms gripping the vertical surface like a spider, her legs spread, knees bent and tense as if she was, at any moment, either going to take flight and run screaming from the room or slide unconscious down the wall. Susan was little better. Her hands, swathed in surgical gloves and bloody, trembled as she continued to hold a liver lobe aside at the spot where I had been working. Her eyes, too, were wide and rimmed with surprise.

I was afraid to look at Elaine. Throughout the ordeal, there had not been a sound from the corner where she stood. I wasn't sure whether that was good news or bad. When I finally summoned the courage to look at her face, I was stunned to find there a serene and untroubled expression of complete calm. Her eyes were soft and steady as they returned my gaze, and though I could not see her mouth under the surgical mask, I was sure she was smiling sweetly. Her hands were clasped comfortably in front of her and she leaned nonchalantly against the wall. I could find not a trace of alarm or concern on her face or in her demeanor.

Her steadiness snapped me quickly back to the task at hand. I had to go through the entire process of scrubbing, gowning, and gloving again before I could proceed with the surgery, but the rest of the procedure was anticlimactic. In short order, I had repaired the hole in the diaphragm, tested for leaks, placed another chest tube, and closed the abdominal wall and skin. In no time at all, we were carrying Max back to his cage and pulling off our masks, gowns, caps, and gloves. Max's recovery after that was rapid and complete. He was ready to go home within two days and was almost back to normal by the time we released him.

It was not until suture-removal time two weeks later that I dared to bring up the incident to Elaine. I asked her if she had been afraid or worried when things started to go wrong, and how she had remained so calm.

"I did notice that the three of you were pretty stressed. But there was nothing whatsoever I could do to help. I was sure you would soon have everything under control. And I figured that the last thing you needed was for me to flip out on you. And I was right to be so confident, wasn't I? Look at him. Max is one hundred percent back to normal. You did a great job!"

I could have hugged her on the spot. How in the world it was that she had witnessed such unadulterated panic in the face of unexpected crisis without losing every shred of confidence in my skills amazes me still as I think about it. I had dodged a bullet!

There was, however, fallout from Max's surgery. Ginny's career as a veterinary assistant did not survive it. From that day on, she vehemently refused to be the anesthetist for surgical patients. Within just a few short weeks, in fact, she left my employment, choosing instead to go to grooming school to master that less stressful aspect of pet care. To this day, Ginny blames Max's surgery for her career change. The terror of it was just too much for her. When she completed her training, she opened a pet-grooming parlor in a nearby community, where she is still a groomer today.

But there were no consequences with Elaine. Now, some ten or twelve years later, she is still a loyal client of mine. Sadly, Megan and Max are now both gone. But Elaine has two new dogs, young, exuberant, and wonderful chocolate Labs. Their pictures are pinned to the message board above my desk. In fact, as I look at the appointment book, I am pleased to see that Elaine has an appointment for both of her new dogs in the morning. I will remain forever grateful to her for her continued friendship and the confidence she still places in me, despite Max's exciting surgery.

FIGHTING THE GOOD FIGHT

There lies within some people an unseen and unseeable reserve of strength and energy, unbelievable optimism in the face of improbable odds, overflowing wells of goodwill, and constantly optimistic attitudes. Some of us are endowed with limitless stores of these qualities, stores which can be requisitioned in times of need — our own or the needs of others — despite the emergence of the burgeoning forces arrayed against us. Others, faced with similar circumstances, or even those not nearly approximating the same harshness, grovel and feign, wrap themselves in layers of excuses and complaints, thereby making their own lives piteous and unbearable, and casting the lot of those around them into deep shadow. Tragedy does not create in a person good character; tragedy only reveals the courage, the integrity, the forbearance, and the inner wellspring of strength that lie quiescent within those whose inner selves are constructed of these raw materials.

Lisa's therapy took on a life of its own. The awful weekly visits and the flushing of toxic medical sludge through an already-ravaged body assumed a sort of routine, as if it was normal, which, for Lisa, it unfortunately had become. Throughout the process, Lisa maintained a positive outlook, calling on stockpiles of courage she had not known she possessed. Most of the time she felt well, despite days when waves of nausea washed over her and crashed into her seawall of resolve and determination. Somehow that wall held. Early on, there were only a few days when she was too ill to come to work, and when she was there, her work was largely unaffected.

For weeks this pattern repeated itself: a round of chemotherapy, followed by illness, doctor's visits, blood work, follow-up MRIs, then another round of chemo. Lisa was placed on antibiotics when her white-blood-cell count dropped; at these times she stayed away from the potentially contagious things to which she might be exposed at the office. The medications helped in large part to keep the creeping nausea at bay, except for a day or two after her treatments. Her hair thinned noticeably but did not completely fall out. She resisted shaving her head, falling back on wearing hats instead.

Despite Lisa's fears, Dave was a constant and ready source of help and support, though I cannot imagine the torment he must have endured in doing so. Steven and Melanie were stalwart in their support, although they were often absent. Steven's assignment in the military prevented him from spending much time at home, though he called often and committed his few free weekends to his mother. Melanie had moved on to a job in New York, the city that never sleeps, where, it seemed, neither did she. Besides Dave, Susan was Lisa's real ally, always ready with a meal, a shoulder, a word. She fed the horses when Lisa could not get out of the house. She ran errands to the pharmacy or the grocery store. She kept Lisa centered at those infrequent times when her mind veered unavoidably toward the morose.

I tried to be available for Lisa, but our daily interactions really didn't change much. They focused mostly on the ongoing flow of animals that eddied around us for treatment or surgery. Occasionally, Lisa asked me for clarification of some misunderstood medical terminology her doctors had used or wanted me to look at the latest

X-ray, but usually the subject of her illness or its treatment was not broached. This left me feeling oddly guilty that I was not doing more for her, but I assuaged that guilt with the hope that if she needed help from me, she would ask. The fact that she had not done so, suggested to me that I was providing for her a sense of the normal, ordinary, mundane flow of "real" life that staked her to her world and allowed moments of blissful forgetfulness of the shadow within.

I discovered a surprising emotional response to the situation when I shared news of Lisa's plight with others. It startled me how often their initial reaction to news of her lung cancer was to ask if she was a smoker. It should not have surprised me. I had done so myself — many times, in fact — when presented with a similar scenario. But from my new perspective as someone intimately connected to the afflicted person, these questions struck me first as insensitive, then as offensive. The intimation was that since Lisa had engaged in such risky behavior, the resultant illness was a foregone conclusion, an expected and therefore an acceptable outcome — as if cancer in a smoker is somehow less tragic. It is true, of course, that smoking is often at the root of lung cancer. But even if a person's poor choices lead to an awful disease, the tragedy for that person is no less intense. The family is still ravaged, the souls still tattered.

This realization was an epiphany for me, one that gained credibility when I learned a few statistics regarding the occurrence of lung cancer in people. I learned, for instance, that 90 percent of lung cancer patients are or have been smokers. This was not a surprise to me. It came, in fact, as a self-righteous confirmation of many long-held assumptions. Serves them right, I would huff, gathering around my shoulders the blankets of assurance that, as a non-smoker, my own chances of a similar diagnosis were minuscule. But the statistics that followed took me off guard. Only 10 percent of smokers develop lung cancer. My first thought was disbelief. Certainly that number was too low. But then doorways of deeper empathy and sensitivity were opened for me, swinging much easier on the hinges of my friendship with Lisa.

Smoking is not an immutable sentence of lung cancer. It is, like any number of other things, just a risk factor for it — a very significant risk factor, to be sure, but nothing more. To assume more is simply an unthinking, self-absorbed response to our own fear of mortality. Though an understandable reaction, it diminishes in our minds the very real catastrophe for the stricken person, a mistake of enormous consequence, for it becomes an unconscious and unintended demonstration of insensitivity.

This perspective is not some macabre defense of smoking in any way. There are reams of documentation linking cancer and a host of other maladies to smoking. High blood pressure, emphysema, coronary artery disease, chronic bronchitis, laryngeal cancer, asthma, and any number of other diseases have been shown unequivocally to be caused by smoking. I have, though, been struck with the realization that to lay the blame on the victims of lung cancer, or these other diseases, is useless and patronizing and compromises our ability to truly empathize with those who find themselves in the position that we most fear. I found myself saying in the face of statistics and risk factors and scientific associations, "Yeah, those are all true. But this is Lisa we're talking about here. She isn't a statistic. She's my friend." It was only at this point that I could really begin to care.

For a time, it appeared that the enemy within Lisa was being beaten back. Lisa's shortness of breath improved, in fact, as did her intolerance to exertion. Even the cough abated for a while. For a few months, it seemed that the war might have been won. But it is often easy to mistake winning a battle with the harder task of victory in the war. After a few months of apparent victory, it was as if the powerful medicines became no more effective than waving flimsy branches at the attacks of a lion, a pride of lions. It became apparent that to continue the feeble offensive was not the height of bravery, but would be instead the foolishness of cowards, afraid to face the certainties of defeat. Lisa was no coward. When the time came to acknowledge that her treatments were not working, she was able to do so with the same strength and resolve with which she had endured them.

The intent of her therapy changed at that point from attempts at cure to efforts at minimizing the impact of her disease. Medications to diminish the intractable discomfort and pain replaced those that inflicted short-term suffering in hopes of long-term resolution. Lisa's interactions with her family began to focus on equipping them for the inevitable; with expressing to them her visions for how she hoped their lives would unfold. She displayed an awareness of issues deeper and more overarching than those to which her day-to-day routines gave voice. I'm sure she must have grappled with the fundamental questions common to us all, but hers were private thoughts. Dave was a source of strength for her, remaining by her side even when she demanded, for his own good, that he desert her.

One evening after work, I drove to Lisa's house and sat down with the two of them. She had asked that I come by to discuss a few details that were important to her. She was completely in control of the discussion that evening, indulging in neither sentimentalism nor self-pity. It is a conversation that I relive with a sense of disbelief, wondering if I could be so endowed with dignity and rationalism if I was presented with similar constraints of time and future. I sat on the edge of an overstuffed chair in her living room, facing the two of them on the couch. Grizzly lay at their feet, looking up at me suspiciously, as if I was there to inflict upon Lisa some of the same insults, injections, and probing I had imposed upon him through the years.

"How are you doing, Lisa?" She knew it was not a casual non sequitur, and she didn't treat it as such.

"For the most part, I'm still doing okay.

But I can tell things are going downhill." She responded with an openness and honesty that smarted. "They tell me that the tumor has spread to my liver and kidneys."

"Have they seen that on MRIs?"

"No, they quit doing those. There's really no point. They can just feel the liver getting bigger. I can, too, if I press a little bit."

"Are you in pain?"

"Not really. The morphine does a pretty good job most of the time."

Dave sat beside her, holding her hand and nodding in agreement and affirmation, seeming no more affected by the articulation of these realities than when they remained an unspoken, although very constant, presence. Expression, in fact, seemed to minimize the impact for both of them. The disease was their abiding companion, having become now a familiar reality. It was a cheerless presence, to be sure, but it was not for them what it was for me: a faceless Evil with whom I was only distantly familiar, the source of a dreadful, unarticulated fear whose confluence I was unaccustomed to confronting.

"Doc, there are a few things I'm going to need your help with from here on out."

"You know I'll do anything I can for you anytime."

"I'm concerned about Grizzly."

I had suspected he would be one of her priorities. He was advancing in age, though not yet truly geriatric. He had been suffering recently from a series of undiagnosed pains. His neck was the source of significant discomfort. To avoid shooting pain, he kept it still and rigid, moving only his eyes instead of his whole head. There was muscle wasting over his hips and shoulders for no apparent reason, as if he was tiring from the chore of carrying the vast weight of Lisa's world. He had developed a grouchy, unpredictable attitude around everyone but Lisa, whom he continued to idolize. I suspected that the degree of her illness and the limits imposed by the physical and emotional trauma of her treatment were not lost on Grizzly, inflicting their toll not on Lisa alone but on this noble and devoted soul, as well.

Jane Goodall has explored the fascinating world of unspoken connections between people and their pets and the inaudible but unimpeachable levels of shared communion between them in her wonderful documentary, *When Animals Talk*. Grizzly's physical manifestations of discomfort, his surprising and uncharacteristic change in personality, his tireless companionship with Lisa, were perfect examples of this physical, emotional, and spiritual union, a passionate iteration of his connection to Lisa's failing body. On his heart came to rest the full weight of the sadness and loss, the unfairness, the pathos, the physical ruin, heedless to entreaties, which Lisa could neither understand nor vocalize.

Grizzly asked for no clarification from Lisa. He knew her heart, not because she had articulated it to him but because he shared it, was a part of it. Two hearts, his and hers, each assigned to separate individuals, were nonetheless one functioning unit. It is this mysterious union of hearts bridging barriers of skin, sinew, and species that is the very substance of the Gift that pets extend to us so generously, so unselfishly. The Gift is a bond between, a contract with, a promise from, and a claim upon two hearts — a circle that encompasses the very essence of those hearts. It is a circle as large as the universe; as small as the molecules of love and devotion that bind together two disparate hearts; a circle that contains all that is vital and alive, into which we can pour every whit of ourselves, unadorned and without fear of judgment or rejection. The circle is as powerful as the unbreakable and eternal bonds of love, as fragile as the cruel whims of temporal brevity and rancorous contagion.

It is the fragile circle in which I thrive; a thousand fragile circles to which I am a servant. They wholly encircle me, yet involve me only tangentially. As a veterinarian, I am a privileged observer of a myriad of such circles, entwining thousands of human and animal hearts. My perspective is intimate and personal, infused with import by its proximity to these circles. Like the circuits described by the orbits of electrons around a nucleus, these fragile circles vibrate with emotional energy and give voice to a fundamental force of the human soul. And now, nearing the time when Lisa knew this circle would have to change shapes and forms, her concern turned to Grizzly, as his had been trained on her.

"What worries you about Grizzly?" I asked quietly.

"When I go, it will be too hard on him. He won't understand. So I'd like you to promise me something. And this is really important to me."

I nodded but did not speak.

"I'd like you to put Grizzly to sleep so he can go with me. I'm not sure whether my family wants me buried or cremated, and it doesn't matter to me. But either way, I want

Grizzly to be with me. Can you do that for me?"

"Yes, Lisa, I can."

"Some of my family may not want it that way. They may want to take Grizzly themselves for the rest of his life. But I'm counting on you and Dave to see that it happens the way I want."

"You have my word on it, Lisa." I was quiet for a moment. "And Zepp?"

"Zepp can live out his days with Mom. He's still a memorial to Steve. And I think he loves Mom."

"I'll take care of Zepp his whole life, Lisa. Don't worry about that."

The story didn't continue much longer after that. Lisa worsened each week. Her last days were spent in the hospital. There remains in my mind an unfading, ineradicable image of Lisa the last time I saw her, only a day or so before she passed. Her family had gathered at the hospital. I greeted Steven and Melanie and Amelia with embraces of sadness and compassion. Then Susan and I entered Lisa's room.

The lights were low and the room was quiet except for the humming of the monitors and fluid pumps. Quiet, that is, except for the constant rasping effort of Lisa's desperate breathing, each breath a mortal battle, one that she would have lost had she lain back restfully on her bed. In order to force the rebellious air into her overrun lungs, she had to sit upright, her face to the ceiling, her mouth open and gasping. I went to her and she gratefully leaned against me. The air she was able to consume was too costly to expend on words, so she just turned her desperate and fearful eyes to me. Yes, there was fear there. Who wouldn't be fearful? Had she done enough? Said enough? Loved enough? Had she prepared her children adequately for the road ahead? There was also fear, perhaps, of the great unknown and unknowable. Lisa had not been a particularly religious person, after all, and had not seemed inclined to indulge those thoughts before. Fear even of the next breath itself, that she might not have the strength, the will to draw it.

Yet there was more than fear in her eyes. Registered in them was also a knowing that I cannot express. There was a knowledge, I presume, that soon the battle would be over, and perhaps there was gratitude for that. A knowledge that the enemy, Cancer, had finally won, a hollow victory for him at this point. There was acknowledgment that her influence in this world would soon cease, that her ability to intercede for her loved ones and to intervene in their affairs was gone. And there was an awareness that despite the attendant pain and loss and parting, life is worth it; that hers had been spent in valuable pursuits that would outlive her.

It is tempting to spend pages drawing life-altering lessons from the story I have unfolded. And I know there are some. I have certainly learned many from it myself. But who am I to point out to you anything other than how the tale has impacted me? I am not learned. I am not a sage or a philosopher. I am only a scribe, the simple teller of the tale and a witness to its truthfulness, though tears even now trace their way from my eyes to your heart. I can write the words with careful craft, but I cannot read them aloud without once more spilling tears. Interpretation is not my task. It is for you to apply the blood to your own doorposts.

Lisa was my friend. And if I could say anything to her now, it would be this. "Your influence did not cease the day your breathing did. You influence me still. I sense it when I take advantage of the training and skills of my present-day technicians. I honor it by recognizing the value of the Gift, the import of the bonds of the fragile circle between my clients and their pets, like the one between you and Grizzly. It is evident even now when Steven brings his children to the office to meet me — your grandchildren. Perhaps it will be disseminated widely with this telling, to impact many more people, unknown to you or me.

"I have kept my promises to you. Zepp, now a senior citizen, still comes to me, brought in by your aging mother, Amelia, her eyes still bearing the weight and sadness of your absence. I have faithfully provided Zepp's veterinary care all these years, cheerfully without charge, in memory of both you and Steve. With tears in my eyes, I personally injected into Grizzly's vein the solution that slipped him through the portal of the fragile circle to join you, figuratively and permanently. I carried him myself into the funeral home, where his remains would join yours, as your hearts had been joined for years.

"And I have done more than I promised. I went to your house, with your mother's permission, and took Tillie's stone from there to the office building, where I placed it under a tree planted in her memory. And if ever I build a new office, I will carry Tillie's stone there, too, placing it under another tree, perhaps outside my office window, where I will be able to see it with just a glance when I think of you, which I still so often do."

THE NUTTY CASE OF GUMBO

Mrs. Adler was a kind white-haired woman about sixty years of age who presented her little poodle, Gumbo, for evaluation of an ongoing problem. She was a thin, proper, and thoroughly pleasant woman who always dressed in smart, fashionable clothes. Though she was reserved and rather shy, it was obvious that Gumbo was the apple of her eye.

She told me how she had adopted Gumbo from a rescue organization as a young adult dog. The two had bonded right away, their close relationship cemented when her husband had passed unexpectedly, leaving her beloved dog as her only companion. She had recently moved with Gumbo from the crush of the northern Virginia population and very much enjoyed the more relaxed atmosphere in the valley.

Because they were new residents in town, I had seen Gumbo and Mrs. Adler on only one or two occasions. Gumbo had been well cared for at his former veterinarian's office. I could follow the course of his medical history in the records that Mrs. Adler brought with her on her first visit. Fortunately for Mrs. Adler, he had already been neutered when she had adopted him years ago, saving her the added expense of the procedure. Since his adoption, Gumbo had been a boringly healthy patient, seen only annually for his routine vaccinations. Mrs. Adler had been religious about making sure Gumbo received his heartworm-preventive medications each month and kept flea and tick medications on him to prevent the many tick-borne diseases.

Gumbo was the epitome of the patient I had always sworn that I would not treat. In high school and college, when asked what my career aspirations were, I would proudly describe my ideal job as that of an equine veterinarian spending my days outdoors or in a truck, working exclusively with horses. "I'd never want to spend my days stuck in some office, working on poodles with painted nails that belong to some little old lady with blue hair," I'd proclaim.

This thought struck me when I first looked at my new patient. Gumbo, as pleasant and well-mannered as his owner, was approximately eleven or twelve years of age and had short-cropped curly white hair. The groomer had fashioned the characteristic topknot on his head and had decorated each ear with a blue bow, held in place with a rubber band. Like many aging poodles, Gumbo had numerous small warts dotting his skin and a hint of gray starting to shade his pupils. His hair was shaved close to the skin on his feet, allowing me to easily see the bright red polish that had been painstakingly applied to Gumbo's nails.

And yet, though Gumbo was exactly the type of dog I'd had in mind when I'd made my pronouncement, the truth was that after almost twenty-five years in small-animal practice, he was now the type of patient I most enjoyed treating. For me, the emotional connection between owners and their pets provides the spark that ignites my work with meaning. It was clear that Gumbo was indeed an honored member of Mrs. Adler's family.

"What seems to be Gumbo's problem, Mrs. Adler?" I asked as I entered the examination room. My initial assessment, as I watched Gumbo circling her legs anxiously, failed to reveal any telltale symptoms. He looked fearfully from her to me and back again, his tail tucked and his ears back.

"You know, it's hard to put my finger on it, really," she responded. "He's just not acting right. He seems antsy — like he's just uneasy all the time. And it seems to be getting worse rather than better. It's just not like him."

"When did you first notice these changes?"

"I suppose it's been two or three weeks."

I nodded my head but automatically added a week or two to her estimate. People almost always underestimate the duration of a problem — especially if it is a chronic one. The more vague the guess, the more time I add. The owners don't do this purposely to throw me off track or to justify their negligence of the problem. They simply tend to forget how long their pets have been dealing with any given issue. But unless they tell me that they first noticed the problem yesterday, I generally add about 50 percent of their guess to the time frame

"Okay, and has he cried out or shown any specific signs of pain?" I asked.

"I can't say that he has; just a general discomfort."

"Any squealing when you lift him or hesitancy to jump on or off the furniture or go up or down the stairs?"

"Yes, he has been hesitant to jump up on

the couch recently, now that you mention it." Mrs. Adler looked at me with a bemused look on her face, as if I had just read her palm. "How did you know that?"

"Just a hunch," I replied. "And has he been slow to move around? Like he's just generally sore?"

"Yeah, that's it. Just achy like."

A clinical picture was emerging from her vague description. It sounded like Gumbo had a sore back. With that in mind, I watched Gumbo move around the room, looking for evidence that he was guarding his back or showed a subtle deficiency of gait or a reluctance to move his back or neck normally. But as he pranced around the room, still nervous and jumpy, I saw no hint of any discomfort. This did not necessarily dissuade me from considering back pain. Often I find that back sufferers, in the stressful environs of a veterinary office, release enough adrenaline to provide temporary relief from their discomfort.

"Why don't we take a look at the little guy, Mrs. Adler," I said, squatting down to lift the eight-pound poodle onto the examination table. Usually I leave the task of lifting small patients to the owners, never sure how they will react. Many dogs, who usually approach me eagerly for a pat on the head or a scratch behind the ears, will react with a surprised nip at my hands when I try to lift them. Once on the table, they usually relax enough to allow me to examine them. But in Gumbo's case, I wanted to see if I could identify any grunt or wince of discomfort at the pressure on his back while being lifted. Again, there was no noticeable reaction.

Once he was on the table, I carefully gave him a thorough examination, focusing in on his back. But despite my suspicions, I could elicit only very subtle discomfort as I pressed on the spine, moving from his pelvis and continuing forward to his neck. Neither could I identify any pain in any of his joints or in his belly. His heart and lungs sounded fine; his temperature was normal. With the exception of this vague discomfort in his back, everything seemed just fine. I turned, puzzled, to Mrs. Adler.

"Well, I'm sure not finding anything convincing on little Gumbo. Perhaps just a tad discomfort over the lower back. But it doesn't seem significant, at least not enough to make him show the signs you describe." I paused, thinking carefully. "I think we should do some blood work to rule out any metabolic problems. As long as the blood work is okay, I'll prescribe some pain medications for a couple of weeks directed at a mild back strain. If things don't get better with that, then we should do some X-rays to see if we can find anything that explains his symptoms."

It took just a matter of a few minutes before I had Gumbo's test results in my hands. They were boringly normal. Early in my career, I felt apologetic if the results of some test were normal, as if I had wasted the client's money by doing a needless test. But experience has taught me that the best news a client can hear is that their pet's tests are normal. It means that I can cross a host of bad diseases off the list of possible diagnoses. Mrs. Adler responded with relief to the results and gladly took two weeks of pain-relieving medications home for Gumbo with instructions to enforce strict rest during that time.

Three or four days later, Mrs. Adler called to report that Gumbo seemed to be acting more like himself. She was pleased with his progress and thanked me for my assistance. Given the good report, I took Gumbo off my mental checklist.

And, of course, there were a million tiny details of practice management that demanded my constant attention. There were decisions to make about whether or not to stock a new medication. There were employee reviews to complete, checks to sign, interpersonal staff dramas to referee. Even such a seemingly insignificant detail as supplying containers large enough to accommodate large tissue samples that needed to be biopsied had to be considered. The pathology laboratory supplied small jars filled with formalin for small samples. But sometimes the growths removed from our patients were too large to fit into these small containers. So a general announcement needed to be made to the staff to bring in jars of varying sizes, in which we could submit larger tissue samples. Details, details. The devil is in the details, they say. And every day is crowded with hundreds of them, it seems.

So it was a surprise to me when a week or two later (or it could have been longer, so add a week to that if you must) I noticed a recheck appointment on the computer for Mrs. Adler and Gumbo. I had to review the record to remind myself of the details of Gumbo's case before I entered the room where the pair had been escorted.

I found Mrs. Adler, beautifully coiffed and dressed sharply in a well-matched outfit of dress slacks and a colorful blouse, with an understated string of simple pearls around her neck and a gold bracelet around her slim wrist, sitting on the bench in the exam room. Her face was pinched and concerned. Gumbo was on the floor in front of her, still and drawn, in as odd a stance as I had seen any patient assume.

His front legs were together in front of him, stretched out, calm and serene, as if his front half was about to nod off for a nice afternoon nap. His back half, though, appeared not to have gotten the same memo. His rear legs were extended straight, raising his hips and pelvis into a position that made me think at any moment he might send his back end running off after a squirrel, leaving his front half in place, still asleep and unconcerned. The effect would have been humorous had it not been evident that this stance was the result of some significant internal discomfort.

"He looks really uncomfortable now, doesn't he?" Mrs. Adler commented unnecessarily. "He did really well for a while after I gave him his course of pain pills. But in the last two days, this is what he does. And he does it all the time. He even does it as he stands at his bowl to eat."

"He's still eating, though, huh?" I observed. "Any vomiting or diarrhea?"

"No, but now he grunts a bit when I lift him. And he just stands around the house in this pose, like he's doing the downward dog yoga position or something."

I lifted him gently onto the table. He responded with an audible grunt and an indignant nip at my hand. My hands went first to his neck and back, where I expected a dramatically painful reaction to the manipulation along his spine. But he remained quiet. His back was not the issue.

When I encircled his tiny abdomen with my fingers and gently felt his tummy, though, a firm tangerine-size lump was immediately detectable. It took up most of the space in his belly, just in front of his back legs. Its bulk took me by surprise. But what was even more startling was Gumbo's frantically excruciating reaction to my gentle squeezing of the mass. He turned to me, a look of surprised offense on his face, and squealed once, loudly.

"Wow, that really hurts!" I said without thinking.

"What is it?" Mrs. Adler turned anxious eyes up to me, her hands covering her ears after the awful shriek of pain.

"There is a large lump in Gumbo's belly that hurts like anything when I squeeze it even the tiniest bit."

"A lump? What, exactly, does that mean?"

"I'm not sure what the lump is yet, but

it's not supposed to be there. We're going to have to do some things to find out. I think the first thing we need to do is an ultrasound of his tummy. If everything else looks okay, then we need to go in surgically and get rid of that lump. And we need to do that right away."

"You have permission to do anything Gumbo needs to make sure he's okay."

Mrs. Adler left the office, and I took Gumbo to the back and had the technicians shave his little belly. I placed the probe of the ultrasound machine on his tummy and watched the shades of gray echoes coalesce to form an image of a large mass in Gumbo's crowded abdomen, pushing his intestines and kidneys to the outer edges. A few twists of my wrist let me evaluate each of the organs. All else appeared normal, with no hint of spread to the liver, spleen, or kidneys. The growth appeared distinct and unattached to other organs. It did not appear to invade or encompass any large blood vessels. That was good. All indications were that whatever it was could be removed surgically.

While the techs prepared Gumbo for the surgery, I went to the phone to report my findings to Mrs. Adler. Gumbo was placed back in his kennel, where he immediately assumed the head-down, tail-up position that I had never seen any other patient exhibit. He maintained this stance even after pain medications and sedatives were administered.

I did not know quite what to expect as I entered Gumbo's belly that afternoon. Once I had opened the abdomen with my scalpel, though, a large reddish purple growth practically jumped through the incision of its own accord. The growth had originated in an undescended testicle; invading it and replacing the normal anatomy with an angry tumor that had grown, unchecked, to enormous proportions. It was a simple thing to place a quick ligature around the engorged blood vessels that fed the ugly growth and to snip them beside the sutures. The whole thing was deposited onto the tabletop within just a few minutes.

A little searching exposed the opposite testicle, only about an eighth the size of its cohort, hiding just behind the kidney. It, too, had failed to migrate from its embryological location down to the scrotum during gestation. Gumbo had never been neutered at all! Since he had come to the rescue organization and Mrs. Adler as a stray, it had been a reasonable assumption to conclude that he had already been under the knife. Unfortunately, retained testicles like Gumbo's have a much higher rate of tumors in them than testicles that descend as nature intended them to.

As a man, my heart went out to this brave little dog, who had been suffering the equivalent of a swift kick to the groin for weeks unending. It was about all I could do to continue to stand at the surgery table to complete the procedure. Only the knowledge that Gumbo would feel better upon recovery from anesthesia than he had for more than a month provided me the necessary fortitude to continue.

Fortunately for Gumbo, most testicular tumors in the dog are benign. Surgical removal, therefore, is usually curative. Still, to be sure this one was benign, it was necessary to send it off for a pathologist to look at microscopically. To be thorough, I directed the technician to include the smaller testicle along with the cancerous one. The size of the mass precluded using one of the small containers that the pathologist provided for such a purpose. I realized this as I watched the technician search through the cabinet in which the miscellaneous jars for oversize biopsies were stored, holding in my hands both the shrunken tiny testicle and the grossly enlarged and angry tumorous one.

As she stood and removed the lid to the jar that she had selected, she unexpectedly broke into a helpless belly laugh that continued with absolutely uncontrollable mirth. Failing to see the humor in the situation, I waited, dumbfounded, and watched her as she continued to guffaw.

"What in the world is so funny?" I asked. Her laughter continued despite the confused look on my face. In response, she stood and turned the label of the jar so I could read it.

It said MIXED NUTS!

THE SUGAR GLIDER

Every profession has its disadvantages, those unpleasant or disturbing tasks that must be done as part of the job. They come with the territory. For veterinarians, it is the all too frequent chore of performing euthanasias. While it is true that these are almost always done in the context of a long-term loving relationship between a heartbroken family and a sick or dying pet, it is an emotionally draining task nonetheless.

On the flip side, every profession also comes with its array of benefits that are available in no other line of work. There are myriads of such positive rewards for me as a veterinarian. Among them are the opportunities to develop long-lasting and meaningful relationships with a host of wonderful families — relationships that often outlast the life span of the first animal I have treated.

I suppose the most exciting professional

perk for me is the chance to see and interact with a huge variety of cases and patients. Not only are the types of cases ever new and exciting but the species of animal continually changes, as well. Mine is perhaps the only profession where a doctor can be presented with a patient that is the first individual of that species he has ever seen. This has happened to me on many occasions, and each time the thought of it has sent shivers of anxiety through me. But it has also always kept my practice fresh and stimulating.

Such was the case the first time I saw a sugar glider. What, you may ask, is a sugar glider? And a good question it is — one that I asked of my receptionist, who was not able to answer the question for me. She came to me one day, asking if I would be willing to see a sugar glider with a tail problem. I told her to tell the caller that I would be more than willing to see a new patient. Then I went straight to my computer, where I looked online at one of the many veterinary forums to learn what I could about the species I was about to treat.

Sugar gliders, it turns out, are small marsupials from Australia and are about the size and shape of a flying squirrel. I read that they are quick, curious, and fun little pets that are gaining surprising popularity for their energy and responsiveness. I was about to find out for myself.

Later that day, I was introduced to Perky, a small brown-and-tan-striped mammal with a pouch like a kangaroo and astonishingly large brown eyes and round ears, weighing in at under half a pound. Most gliders have a full, thick, and ever-active bushy tail, which provides balance and is a failsafe barometer of their attitude. Perky's, though, bent almost double on itself about an inch from its tip and hung, sadly still, beyond that spot.

Even with an obviously injured tail, Perky was a bundle of nonstop activity, climbing up and down his owner's torso with bursts so rapid that it was almost difficult to see his little legs moving. Despite the hanging chad of a tail tip, he still flicked his tail when I entered the room, making it clear, even to one who had never seen the species before, that my presence stressed him. Sugar gliders are beautiful and incredibly engaging little animals, and I was immediately enthralled by him.

"He's the most beautiful sugar glider I have ever seen. We don't see many of these, so I don't know that much about the species," I said. The first sentence was absolutely true. The second obfuscated the fact that I knew absolutely nothing about them. "Are they gentle?"

"Perky is really gentle with people," said Jeanie, a tall, pleasant woman in her late twenties who was wearing a T-shirt and jeans. "I have five gliders, and Perky is by far the friendliest."

With that endorsement, I reached over and snatched the little squirmer from Jeanie's back, where he was surveying me with wide, intense eyes. Without a moment's hesitation, he turned and bit me on the finger — not hard enough to draw blood but enough so that my reaction was to jerk my hand away, sending him flying onto the tabletop. Clients always seem to derive sadistic pleasure from any pain their pets inflict upon the doctor. Jeanie was no exception. Laughing appreciatively, she reached toward the tabletop to pick up the little nipper. Perky dodged her and jumped instead onto her shirt again, running around to the side farthest away from me, like a squirrel circling a tree trunk.

"They do tend to nip a bit," Jeanie said unnecessarily. "You've just got to expect it. Luckily, they don't bite hard. It's mostly just a surprise when they get you."

"Well, it sure did surprise me," I responded. In the few seconds I had held the glider, I was amazed at the whipping-cream softness of his dense coat and how light he was in my hand. I had expected there to be more substance to him, but he was only a few ounces of mostly soft fur. "What happened to his tail?"

"I really don't know. He was fine when I put him in his cage for the evening. But when I came to get him this morning, his tail was like that. I think he's broken it."

"It sure looks like it. But I'll need to get him to stay still long enough for me to feel it before I'll know for sure."

I reached and grasped the glider again, this time by the scruff, on the assumption this would allow me to control his mouth. It is a technique that works like magic with fractious cats. For the record, though, it doesn't work at all for sugar gliders! The scruff was so loose that the little devil was able to turn with his skin still in my grasp and bite me again, this time on the base of my thumb. I did not let go. Fortunately, this time he did. There was hardly room for me to use two hands on him, but two hands were what it took to still him enough for me to feel quickly up and down the length of his tail.

There could be no doubt that the tail was

broken. At the spot of the bend, I could feel the stump of a bone end poking into the skin. There was also a spot of blood left on my finger after palpating the injury — a compound fracture. Surprisingly, Perky hardly reacted to my probing, though I'm sure it must have been painful. His only response was to turn and sink his little teeth into my hand again the instant I released him.

Gamely, I grabbed the little demon again. My enchantment with the species was waning in proportion to the number of times Perky had tagged me. And Jeanie had said he was an especially friendly glider! I placed my stethoscope on his heaving little chest. The head of the scope was so large, it covered his entire left side. His heart was racing at a speed I could not count — probably over 350 beats a minute. He turned and bit again, but this time he latched onto my stethoscope.

With gentle fingers, I probed his tummy next. But his torso was too small for me to be able to differentiate internal structures. Besides, in an instant he had turned and bitten me a fourth time on the finger. I had examined everything I was able to, so I let the little animal jump back over onto Jeanie's shirt.

I had to give the animal its due. I had handled him a total of less than a minute and already he had bitten me four times — five if not for one poorly aimed attempt. That was one bite every fifteen seconds. No other animal had ever been that successful in prosecuting their aggressive tendencies with me. It was true that the bites did not seem malicious. They were more Perky's inquisitive attempts to explore the bound-aries and assess the resolve of the white-coated monster who was annoying him. Nor did they hurt that much. Really, they were just a nuisance and an insult to me, when I meant him no harm. But the habit was not one that endeared him to me. In fact, with four bites in rapid succession, this machine gun–like biting menace flat ticked me off.

"So, is it broken?"

"No question about it. And it's a com-pound fracture, too," I responded. "But as active as he is, there is simply no way to stabilize the tail enough for it to heal. He'd never tolerate a bandage or cast of any kind."

"I expect you'll just have to take it off, right?"

"I don't see any other way around it. We can't leave the tail like it is. And we can't repair it. I think the only option is to snip it off. He'll still have enough of a tail that neither you nor he will miss it much."

"Can you do that today?"

"Yes, it shouldn't take too long. Why don't you leave him with me and pick him up later in the day."

I placed Perky in his little transport cage and took him to the treatment room. I would not be able to administer any intravenous drugs to him because of his size and explosive activity level. Instead, I slid his whole head into a mask, through which I pumped oxygen and isoflurane, an anesthetic gas. Isoflurane is a wonderfully safe and effective gas that can be used to anesthetize most anything. Within a minute or less, the frantic struggling of the tiny legs stilled and the breathing slowed. Carefully, I dissected the end of the broken vertebra free from the overlying skin and snipped it off, leaving enough skin to place two quick sutures to close the wound over the stump. The whole procedure was completed in less than three minutes.

Then the excitement began! I pulled Perky's head out of the anesthetic mask and watched for the respiratory movements of his chest wall. There were none. I felt a cold sweat pop up on my face. I reached with my fingers and felt the chest wall for the heartbeat. Though I felt no heartbeat with my fingers, I did feel my own pulse rise as panic began to set in. The mantra of one of my veterinary school professors flashed instantly through my mind: "In an emergency, take your own pulse first." Mine was definitely rapid at that moment.

I snatched the inert form up in my hands, inserted his mouth and nose between my lips, and gave him several quick, short bursts of air, feeling his little chest rise as I did so. With my fingers, I quickly administered a few chest compressions before repeating the artificial respiration. With a wave of relief, I felt Perky's body stiffen and his legs give a quick jerk.

How that animal went from dead to running around the treatment room in less than ten seconds, I will never know. But before I knew it, he had jumped from my hands onto the surgery table and then climbed under the stainless-steel grate covering the sink. I had to throw a towel over him like a fishnet to gain enough control to place him back in his carrier, pleased with myself for successfully bringing him back from the clutches of death.

But my revelry was short-lived. No sooner had Perky been placed back into his carrier than he turned his attention to the tip of his now-shorter tail. In the span of ten seconds, he had snipped the sutures with his sharp incisors. With nothing now closing the wound, his obsessive licking quickly opened it enough so that it started bleeding.

I scooped him up again and replaced his head in the anesthetic mask. When his movements slowed, I quickly placed a couple drops of tissue glue onto the tip of his tail and held the wound closed until the glue had sealed. I then had my technician apply pressure on the tail tip until Perky had once again woken up enough to scamper out of her grasp and back into his carrier.

The glue seemed to stymie him. It was clear that the shortened tail held a fascination for him, since he immediately pulled the amputated stump up to his mouth and licked at it. Fortunately, the glue must have had a bad taste because, though he tentatively tasted it, he did not open the wound again. Putting a makeshift Elizabethan collar on him was out of the question. He was simply too amped to tolerate such an indignity.

And that was my first introduction to the highly charged and caffeinated world of sugar gliders. In the course of one short interaction, I had been introduced to a new species, been bitten by it four times in one minute, anesthetized it twice, performed an amputation on it requiring two methods of surgical closure, and successfully resuscitated it with mouth-to-mouth respirations and chest compressions. I was exhausted.

Perky, on the other hand, seemed none the worse for wear. He went home that night, and though his tail was shorter, he seemed as eager for trouble as he had been when he came in. The Energizer Bunny has nothing on sugar gliders. Cats are supposed to have nine lives. I was not sure how many lives sugar gliders are given. At least one of Perky's had been consumed that afternoon. As for me, the stress of the afternoon came pretty close to exhausting my own supply. I do know that the stress of treating that sugar glider took a toll on me. Sure, variety is the spice of life, but sometimes spices can get just a little too hot!

Denouement

Lisa's passing left us weak and drained. So much emotion had been invested in the process, so much energy in the fight. So much had been stolen by the disease and its treatment. So unfair had been the indifferent election of Lisa by Death himself, piled, as it were, on top of the other sweeping inequities Lisa had known. It was just too difficult to explain to two remaining orphans and a grieving mother; too overwhelming on the tenuous emotions of the reeling team of people in the office. The loss was too much to contemplate, too much to accept.

Lisa's funeral came and went, and still the sheering strain of grief persisted. My mind fought against the enormity of the loss. Surely, I thought, there must be something productive, something meaningful that will emerge from the aching chasm of sadness and frustration left by Lisa's death. But nothing came to me except new waves of sadness.

Dave, apparently, experienced some of the same thoughts. Unlike me, Dave had more motivation. Three or four weeks after Lisa died, he came to me with the idea of establishing a scholarship in her honor at the college where she had trained to become a veterinary technician. A few quick phone calls to the school provided the details of how to go about getting such a fund started. We learned that a permanently endowed scholarship could be established in Lisa's memory with a principal amount of ten thousand dollars. We could have five years to build the fund to that amount. But if the minimum endowment of ten thousand dollars was not reached in that five-year span, the money donated would be awarded in scholarships only until the principal was exhausted.

By putting up signs in the lobby of the hospital, we were able to collect in the first months a few hundred dollars from clients whose pets had benefited from Lisa's skills. Staff members contributed several hundred dollars more. The bulk of the funds contributed came from Dave and from the hospital, which pledged a sizable donation each year for five years.

But as time went on, it became clear that

the ten-thousand-dollar figure would not be reached. Life for others had continued after Lisa's had been truncated, and the flow of time had carried Lisa's memory from the loud, tumbling rapids of frenetic action to the slow-moving, deeper, and more shadowed backwaters of nostalgia, where fondness is sweet but quiescent. The momentum for the scholarship waned, and in the fifth year of the campaign, I received a letter from the college, informing me that the languishing moneys in Lisa's scholarship fund would not be enough for a permanent memorial. I let a long sigh of regret whistle through my lips as I read it. It seemed that, once again, Lisa's potential had been squandered.

Life in the office moved on, as well. There were still patients to be seen and animals to be helped. Plunging headlong into work — in my case, the fray of animal illness — helps to dim the effects of emotion, even emotion intensely felt, and my own and the emotions of the staff subsided with time. New people joined the team after Lisa was no longer there. New receptionists, a new technician or two, new assistants, and even a new veterinarian joined the team. They came and went according to the whims of their circumstances. Many of them contributed greatly to the efficiency of the team and the care of the patients and developed interesting and moving personal stories of their own.

One of the new team members was Krystal Finns. Krystal first joined the staff as a receptionist. She was fairly young, one of the few people I hired soon after she had graduated from high school. She was pleasant and eager, though a bit shy and unsure of herself at first. She had dark hair and eyes and a self-deprecating humor, which accentuated her lack of confidence. I was not sure at first if Krystal would be able to manage the rigors of being a receptionist. Receptionists must be polite and engaging while at the same time maintaining a thick skin and proactive control of their environment. They must be confident in their dealings with a fickle public and have a backbone of steel to handle the onslaught of indifferent and sometimes rude people in a hurry to attend to their companions. They must be clever and witty and armed with an intimate familiarity with a broad range of animal minutiae with which to answer an amazing array of questions. I wasn't sure Krystal, with her inherent shyness, could master these tasks.

But she surprised me. As her training

progressed, she demonstrated a remarkable ability to deal with all kinds of people, putting them at ease in emotionally stressful situations. She quickly learned the information about the patients that made her credible to clients and invaluable to the practice. Her skills with the computer and her grasp of the functions of the office made her the go-to person when technical glitches arose with the computers or the accounting systems in the office. And as time went on, it became clear that Krystal possessed a gift with the animals, as well.

There is an evolution that takes place in many veterinary hospital team members. When someone is hired as a receptionist, it takes some six or eight months to learn the role thoroughly. By the time the person becomes proficient at the task, she develops an interest in the medical aspects of the work that we do and the animals we treat. Inevitably, this evolves into a desire to move into the role of a veterinary assistant. This, I suppose, is natural and to be encouraged. But it creates a constant flow of personnel from one role to another and leaves a frequent hole in the receptionist pool that requires filling.

Krystal soon began to show signs of disquiet in her role as a receptionist and approached me about becoming an assistant. When a need arose for an assistant, I moved Krystal to the position. In this role, too, she showed similar prowess in learning the tasks and quickly became indispensable.

There was another reason Krystal became a popular member of the staff. We quickly learned that, as an only child, she possessed an amazing power over her parents. This power, though she did not display the typical characteristics of a spoiled child, made it possible for doughnuts, pizza, and other such goodies to materialize in the break room when Krystal placed a quick phone call to her mother.

I suppose it was inevitable that Krystal would take the next step of evolution for a veterinary hospital team member. Just about the time she had become invaluable as an assistant, she approached me with a new goal. She wanted to go to school to become a technician. This, too, was predictable. Over the years, I have seen the same progression in no fewer than five or six other employees who have gone back to school to complete their vet-tech training.

Krystal had it all planned out. Her parents were willing to help with the cost of books and gas for the ninety-minute round-trip daily. Her boyfriend had a good job that would support most of their living expenses, though she would still need to work part-time at the office. And tuition would be covered by student loans and a little help from her parents. It would be a sacrifice financially, but she had decided to make it work.

I was proud of Krystal. She had identified her passion and was taking steps to turn her avocation into a vocation. I knew she would be a very good technician, just as she had been a good receptionist and assistant. It would be difficult for her, but she had demonstrated an ability to complete difficult tasks already, and I knew she would be successful. I wrote a glowing recommendation to include with her application and then waited to hear the results. Krystal was as sure she would not be accepted into the program as I was sure of the opposite. I was not surprised to hear in June that she would be entering school in the fall. Krystal was excited, but edging her enthusiasm was a palpable fear, almost a dread, as the fall term approached.

When school started, I discovered the reason for her fear. For Krystal, school had never come as easily as learning the myriad tasks in the hospital had. She was one who excelled at hands-on learning, but she struggled with taking copious notes, reading textbooks, and taking tests. The stress that these activities built in her was evident as she came to work in the evenings. Fortunately, in the office she could see how the facts she was learning applied to actual cases in the hospital, and this connection to real patients grounded her classroom learning.

Then one evening I noticed that Krystal's demeanor was suddenly and decidedly sullen. I was immediately concerned about her academic status, until she confided that her boyfriend had lost his job. This threw their finances into disarray and threatened her ability to continue in the vet-tech program. She was heartbroken as she contemplated the death of her dream. I tried to console her with platitudes about how things would work out and allow her to continue, but my words rang hollow.

Krystal slogged through her first semester with rising panic about how she would afford the tuition once the semester had ended. Though she still performed her clinical duties well, I noticed diminishing enthusiasm about her studies and a strikingly pessimistic approach to her future. Her grades began to dip.

Just before the semester ended in December, there was a sudden change in her attitude and Krystal became the same exuberant person she had been before. I was unsure of the reason for this change until a day or two later as I was opening the mail. Among the bills and the odd Christmas card from an appreciative client was a formal-looking letter with the logo of the community college where Krystal was a student. It was addressed to me, and I opened it with interest.

Inside was a letter that thanked the hospital for its commitment to donations toward the Lisa Spalding Scholarship fund and proudly announced the first recipient of a sizable scholarship awarded to a deserving student in the technician-training program. The first student to receive the scholarship would be Krystal Finns. The scholarship would make it possible for Krystal to remain in the program.

There was a catch in my throat as I held the letter in my hands and reread it quickly. Memories of Lisa flooded my thoughts: the utter transformation of a young girl from quivering insecurity into a settled woman of education, skill, and accomplishment; the sadness of a malignant diagnosis in a person so young; the months of wasting illness, of frantic treatment, and of noble acceptance.

All of this sped through my consciousness. But for the first time, there was also a sense of justice, accomplishment, and completion. Not that Krystal's benefiting from the Lisa Spalding Scholarship was worth the sacrifice. A thousand times no! But something of value had emerged from a story so bleak and sad. I knew how pleased Lisa would be that, as a consequence of the pain she had endured, someone had been able to carry on in the calling that had been life-transforming for her. The fact that it had first benefited someone in Lisa's own practice was icing on the cake, a completion of the circle of yet another story.

Since that time, I have received several additional letters announcing recipients of the Lisa Spalding Scholarship. I suppose at some point the initial moneys contributed will run out and the scholarships will end. But each time I feel much the same satisfaction as I did when Krystal's academic career was salvaged by the scholarship awarded in Lisa's name.

There is something profoundly significant about the completion of this circle; something intensely personal about the scholarships themselves. Though they are no doubt appreciated by the recipients, the true significance, I suppose, is lost on them.

These scholarships represent more than just a windfall from a fund named after some anonymous decedent. For me, they are a nod to a friend; an acknowledgement of a shared passion; an honor to a fallen comrade in the fight for animals; an affirmation that a life was worthy and valuable and well spent even though it was abbreviated. Not everyone's memory is sustained by such noble things, but Lisa's is. Each Christmas, someone who shares her gift and her calling benefits from this award established in her name. It is not enough, of course. But for me, it is of great significance. The Lisa Spalding Scholarship contributes just enough resolution to Lisa's story to season the ache of bitter nostalgia.

A New Home

The clinic constructed when I first opened
the hospital was perfectly suited for one
doctor and the three or four people I needed
to assist me at the time. When the need
arose for me to add a second doctor some
six or seven years later, I was able to reno-
vate the space, adding an examination
room, a break room, and a couple of offices
to accommodate the extra people. But when
the clientele grew to a point where four doctors were needed, the building was just too
small. It had only eighteen hundred square
feet of clinical space, into which I had
crammed three exam rooms, a postage
stamp–size waiting room, a hallway that
doubled as a laboratory, a tiny treatment
room, a surgery room that could accommodate only one table, and a minuscule
X-ray room. The lot was so small that no
room was available to enlarge the building's
footprint, and the parking lot allowed only

twelve spaces. My staff and I were forced to park along the street.

For far too long, I ignored the space constraints, until one day when an emergency patient requiring immediate surgery once again postponed the scheduled surgeries and hurled our day into chaos. It struck me that this could not go on indefinitely, and I was forced, against my will, to consider the construction of a new office building.

For months, Cynthia and I struggled with the decision, spending hours looking over the incredible capital investment this would require. Few people understand the significantly higher financial demands that exist for veterinarians compared to physicians. Setting up an office for us entails more than just a few examination rooms and a nurse or two. We cannot refer our patients next door to the hospital for diagnostic services. We must provide all those functions ourselves. So constructing a new veterinary facility must, by law, include the space and equipment for surgery suites, radiology functions, a laboratory, a pharmacy, hospital wards, and the trained personnel to man them. So considering a new hospital was a mammoth investment.

In the end, the decision was made for us

when we recognized that the overcrowded conditions in the hospital were simply not sustainable. As time went on, we feared that we might well be charged as accessories to murder if we didn't give our staff a bit more elbow room. We began to look for land in town on which to construct a new building.

In such a small community, this had to be done under the cloak of anonymity to prevent the rumor mill from whirling out of control. Most of our search was done simply by driving around the area, looking for land that might be ideal, whether or not it was listed for sale, and then making covert calls to real estate agents or trips to the courthouse to look up who the owners of the property were.

The lot that we settled on was being offered by the state power company, whose real estate overseers were three hours away in Richmond, a fact that worked to our benefit. When the survey revealed that the portion of their land they were willing to sell had no access to the road, the power company was ready to call off the deal. Through some last-minute negotiating with the owners of the land next door, we were able to secure a small triangle of their land that allowed access to the land-locked plot.

Since these maneuvers took over a year to

complete, plans for the building were finished by the time the deal finally occurred. Jace and I had spent many hours tracing out floor plans for the office. Nothing like fourteen years of living with design flaws in one building to inspire a vision for a new space. The company we hired to design and build the office took our hand-scrawled plans, changed them to meet building codes, and returned to us detailed blueprints of a building that was my dream office. I would roll out the plans on our dining room table, spending hours poring over them, envisioning traffic flow, work patterns, and the best way to format the laboratory or position adequate storage. It was intoxicating to plan and dream.

The nine or ten months during construction were exciting times. To see the office take shape, growing out of a vision in my head into something tangible, was great fun, but it was also exhausting. Details like paint colors, tile selection, waiting room furniture, and countertop design took up enormous reserves of time and energy. Weekly meetings with the contractor and subcontractors kept the process moving despite the inevitable unexpected developments.

Our enthusiasm was diminished by reality only on the day of the closing, when our signatures were required on the legal documents that committed us to ungodly payments for years to come. Even that, though, could not dampen our excitement for long.

In the end, we were proud to unveil a state-of-the-art hospital boasting six examination rooms, a spacious treatment room, a surgical suite that would accommodate three surgical tables, a special-procedures room, and a beautiful waiting room for our clients. We more than tripled our clinical space and greatly improved the facilities for our patients, our boarders, our staff and doctors, and the groomer who works with us. We were positioned on three lovely acres at the center of commerce in the community, with room to expand in the future if necessary.

Moving day was a carefully orchestrated event with more tasks than we could accomplish in one day. We closed the hospital for three days, discharging all the patients and boarders, so we would not have to move animals, too. Each staff member was assigned specific tasks. Some had even invited houseguests to help with the move. Early in the morning on the day of the move, we gathered in the tiny break room in the lower level of the old office building to coordinate our efforts.

I don't know what it was about the gathering that stimulated my nostalgia that morning, but I began to remember the accumulation of events in that building that had led to this day. I recalled the details of purchasing the land and building the office; of hiring my first two employees; of long hours spent bent over the surgery table in the tiny surgery room, tediously repairing nasty injuries. I remembered noble patients lost, loyal clients served, and dedicated staff members who had selflessly committed their best efforts to the work. I thought, with sadness, about Lisa and wished she was sitting with us. She would have been so proud of our accomplishments. I thought of Tilley, whose stone was under a tree on the west side of the building, and of Cy, whose stone was under another tree on the east side.

As these thoughts swirled around in my head, I couldn't resist the urge to share them with the staff. They indulged my nostalgia very well, smiling at the memories they shared with me. A few of them even let a tear or two slide down their cheeks with me as we remembered. Then as a group, we made our way outside to the two trees, where we ceremoniously pulled up Tilley's and Cy's marker stones. They would go with us, of course — the very first things moved.

Cy's stone now sits under a tree in the front of the new office. Few of our current clients remember now how she used to sit sphinxlike on the reception desk, welcoming people into the office, her one good eye surveying the patients as they filed nervously into the lobby. Even among the staff, there are now only a few who still hold memories of her — just Susan, Rachel, Cynthia, and me, in fact. And yet for me, her memory encompassed the essence of what had made a new building necessary. The same compassion and devotion to the animals that had saved Cy from the destiny that awaited her had been lavished on our other patients. Of course Cy's stone would make this move with us. Placed with appropriate ceremony in a place of honor, it provided an emotional cornerstone for the new building; CY — EVERYONE'S FRIEND.

And Tilley's stone, too, made the transition from the old building to the new. It sits below a tree just outside my office window, where I can see it as I write records. It is a tribute not only to a courageous dog but to Lisa's memory, and it is also a testament to the many dedicated staff members who, like Lisa, gave their very best to all those patients that made their way through our office, infusing our work with compassion, meaning, and humanity. It remains a reminder to me of the emotional and compassionate intertwining of hearts and hands, of science and souls, of lighthearted laughter and wrenching sadness that form the core of a veterinary hospital. Yes, it is a business, but one that enfolds within its mission the very essence of the fabric woven of the bond between individuals of different species.

It is indeed a Gift to experience this bond — a Gift that has been graciously bestowed on me as it had been on Lisa. But it is also a Gift to be the guardian of this bond, to be charged and entrusted with its protection and maintenance by people wholly consumed by it. This Gift, this magical and all-encompassing treasure, is at the heart of being a veterinarian. And it is a Gift that, for me, has offered untold rewards of love, of fulfillment, of joy and contentment. It has had its challenges, to be sure, but nothing could have provided me with a more wonderful life's work than this. I know if Lisa were here to look with me at Tilley's stone outside my office window, she would agree.

ABOUT THE AUTHOR

Bruce R. Coston, D.V.M., is a winner of the Department of Small Animal Clinic Sciences Service Award. He lives with his family in Virginia.

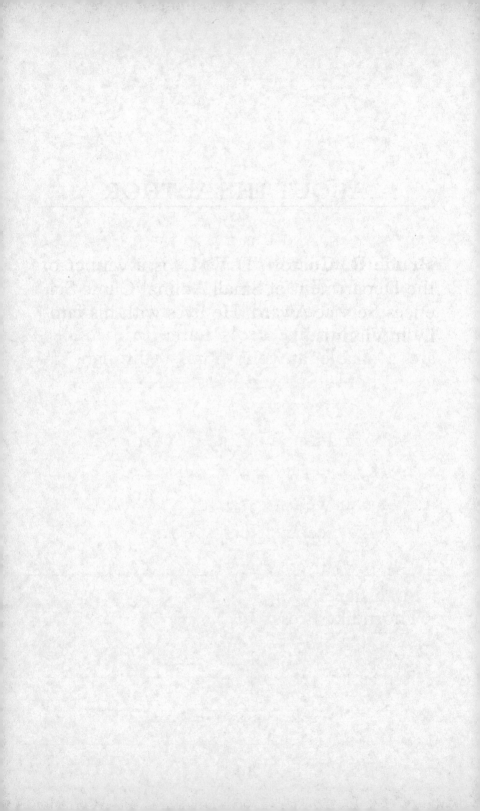